THE NEW PHONOLOGIES

Developments in Clinical Linguistics

THE NEW PHONOLOGIES

Developments in Clinical Linguistics

Edited by

MARTIN J. BALL, Ph.D.

School of Behavioural and Communication Sciences
University of Ulster at Jordanstown
Newtownabbey, Northern Ireland

RAYMOND D. KENT, Ph.D.

Department of Communicative Disorders
University of Wisconsin
Madison, Wisconsin

SINGULAR PUBLISHING GROUP, INC.
SAN DIEGO · LONDON

Singular Publishing Group, Inc.
401 West "A" Street, Suite 325
San Diego, California 92101-7904

Singular Publishing Ltd.
19 Compton Terrace
London N1 2UN, U.K.

e-mail: singpub@mail.cerfnet.com
Web site: http://www.singpub.com

© 1997 by Singular Publishing Group, Inc.

Typeset in 10/12 Palatino by SoCal Graphics
Printed in United States of America by McNaughton and Gunn

Library of Congress Cataloging-in-Publication Data

The new phonologies : developments in clinical linguistics / edited by
    Martin J. Ball & Raymond D. Kent.
      p.   cm
    Includes bibliographical references and index
    ISBN 1-56593-082-7
    1. Articulation disorders.   2. Grammar, Comparative and general—
Phonology.   I. Ball, Martin J.   II. Kent, Raymond D.
    [DNLM: 1. Phonetics.   2. Speech Disorders—physiopathology.
3. Speech-Language Pathology—methods.   WV 501 N532 1997]
RC424.7.N49   1997
616.85'5—DC21
DNLM/DLC
for Library of Congress

96-53434
CIP

Contents

Preface

This book has a twofold purpose. The first is to summarize some of the more recent developments in phonological theory. Phonology is in a highly active phase. Several new theories have been advanced, and modifications of earlier theories have been made. The intellectual pace has been sufficiently brisk that it can be difficult to follow these activities, especially for persons who have an interest in phonology but may specialize in related fields.

The second purpose is to consider the clinical significance of the newer phonologies. Certainly, phonological theories have an intrinsic value as they give us a deeper and more effective understanding of the role of phonology in human language. But these theories also can have worth in applied fields such as speech-language pathology or clinical linguistics and phonetics. The clinical discipline of speech-language pathology frequently has borrowed ideas, concepts, and theories from linguistic studies. Chomsky and Halle's classic book, *The Sound Pattern of English*, was read by many clinicians and by many clinical scientists. Its exploration of lawful patterns in the sounds of a language stimulated a parallel effort in the study of phonological development and phonological disorders. The newer phonologies may bring valuable insights into how phonology is acquired and how it may be disordered. The intent of the book is to suggest ways in which these newer phonologies may influence clinical understanding.

It is hoped that the chapters in this book will provide an effective introduction to the respective theories for readers who want information on the rapidly changing character of phonology. Readers will find between two covers a general introduction to generative phonology, natural phonology, nonsegmental phonology, dependency phonology, grounded phonology, gestural phonology, and optimality theory. The reference lists in each chapter will guide readers to more extensive discussions. In keeping with the second purpose described above, efforts also have been made to point to areas of clinical relevance. But the interest in seeking clinical implications is not simply one directional. Certainly, it is beneficial if these theories can help to guide clinical assessment and intervention. But it is also possible, if not likely, that information from clinical studies can influence theorizing about phonology. One kind of influence is that clinical phonology can help in efforts to develop more constrained phonologies. Another influence is that information on disorders can provide insights that may not be immediately evident in the study of normative phonological behavior. On occasion, the breakdowns of a process can reveal much about the nature of that process. Some breakdowns may mirror patterns in typical development, so that disorders and development are two ways of examining the dynamics of phonology. Another influence is that data on disordered phonologies complement the data on normal phonology. Ideally, a phonological theory should account for both types of data.

We thank the authors who contributed to this volume for their cooperation, patience, and, above all, their expertise.

Contributors

Professor Martin J. Ball
School of Behavioural and
Communication Sciences
University of Ulster at
Jordanstown
Newtownabbey, Co Antrim
Northern Ireland

Professor Pamela Grunwell
Department of Human
Communication
De Montfort University
Scraptoft Campus
Leicester, UK

Professor David Ingram
Department of Linguistics
University of British Columbia
Vancouver, B.C. Canada

Dr. Barbara Handford Bernhardt
School of Audiology and Speech
Science, University of British
Columbia,
Vancouver, B.C. Canada

Professor Daniel A. Dinnsen
Department of Linguistics
Indiana University
Bloomington, Indiana
USA

Professor Raymond D. Kent
Department of Communicative
Disorders
University of Wisconsin
Madison, Wisconsin
USA

Dr. Joseph Stemberger
Department of Communication
Disorders
University of Minnesota
Minneapolis, Minnesota

Professor Carol Stoel-Gammon
Department of Speech and
Hearing Sciences
University of Washington
Seattle, Washington
USA

CHAPTER

1

Introduction: Phonetics for Clinical Phonologies

MARTIN J. BALL AND RAYMOND D. KENT

This book is an introduction to a variety of current phonological approaches to the analysis of the sound systems of language and a demonstration of how they can be applied to disordered speech. In clinical phonology as much as in the phonological analysis of natural language, however, there is one basic prerequisite: a good phonetic description. A phonological theory, however sophisticated its approach or clinically relevant its output, may not help the speech-language pathologist plan remediation, if it is based on faulty phonetic input. As recently described by Ball, Rahilly, and Tench (1996), there are a variety of problems that may result from an oversimplified or inaccurate phonetic analysis of disordered speech data, and we explore a few these here. Examining one of the first examples, one can see the danger of assuming (because of the inaccurate transcription) a neutralization in the client's speech that has not taken place.

The following sample adapted from Ball et al. is given first in broad transcription; as all these transcriptions are nonphonemic (disordered speech by its nature does not conform to a target phonology), square brackets are used throughout. It is noted below which transcriptions are

broad and which narrow (although this is, to some extent, obvious from
the amount of detail included).

Speaker A. Age 7;3. Broad transcription.

shop	[ʃɑːp]	shoe	[ʃuː]
see	[ʃiː]	seat	[ʃiːt]
ship	[ʃɪp]	wash	[wɑːʃ]
sip	[ʃɪp]	yes	[jeʃ]
rush	[ɹʌʃ]	kiss	[kɪʃ]
cushion	['kʊʃən]	messy	['meʃi]

This sample appears to be a clear example of the loss of phonological
contrast between two target phonemes of English: /s/ and /ʃ/, with [ʃ]
being used for both in all places of word structure. Indeed, the minimal pair "sip" and "ship" are in the sample and appear to show a
homonymic clash in speaker A's speech. However, this is a broad transcription, with the transcriber restricting the symbol set to those normally encountered in the transcription of adult target English phonology. This has led to an inaccurate recording of the pronunciation. If we
look at a narrower transcription of the same data with other IPA symbols utilized, a different picture emerges:

Speaker A. Age 7;3. Narrow transcription.

shop	[ʃɑːp]	shoe	[ʃuː]
see	[çiː]	seat	[çiːt]
ship	[ʃɪp]	wash	[wɑːʃ]
sip	[çɪp]	yes	[jeç]
rush	[ɹʌʃ]	kiss	[kɪç]
cushion	['kʊʃən]	messy	[(meçi]

Once this transcription is examined, it is seen that in fact this speaker
has *not* lost the contrast between target /s/ and /ʃ/. It is true that they are
not realized in the standard way, but although [ç] is not a phoneme of
English, and will sound extremely odd being used for /s/, homonymic
clashes do not result from this pronunciation, and so the contrast
between words will not be lost.

   This first example from Ball et al. (1996) involved a major simplification of the transcription process in the broad version, in that the difference between a post-alveolar and a palatal fricative should be quite
noticeable, and is lost in the transcription simply because the transcriber
used only the English consonant symbol set. The authors give a further

example where the phonetic difference is not so great, but the importance of narrow transcription is equally clear.

Speaker B. Age 6;9. Broad transcription.

pin	[pɪn]	ten	[ten]
bin	[pɪn]	den	[ten]
cot	[kɑːt]	pea	[piː]
got	[kɑːt]	bee	[piː]

This data set also suggests that there is a collapse of phonological contrast: specifically the contrast between voiced and voiceless plosives in word-initial position. This clearly leads to homonymic clashes between, for example, "pin" and "bin" and "cot" and "got", respectively. As word-initial plosives have a high functional load in English, such a loss of the feature contrast [±voice] in this context clearly requires treatment. It would appear from these data that an initial stage of treatment would concentrate on the establishment of the notion of contrast with these sounds, before going on to practice the phonetic realization of this contrast.

However, if a narrow transcription of the same data is examined, the picture alters.

Speaker B. Age 6;9. Narrow transcription.

pin	[pʰɪn]	ten	[tʰen]
bin	[pɪn]	den	[ten]
cot	[kʰɑːt]	pea	[pʰiː]
got	[kɑːt]	bee	[piː]

Again, it is clear from this transcription that there is not, in fact, a loss of contrast between initial voiced and voiceless plosives. Target voiceless plosives are realized without vocal fold vibration (voice), but with aspiration on release (as are the adult target forms). The target voiced plosives are realized without aspiration (as with the adult forms), but also without any vocal fold vibration. It is this last difference that distinguishes them from the target form. For, although adult English "voiced" plosives are often devoiced for some of their duration in initial position, totally voiceless examples are rare.

Ball et al. note that although insufficiently narrow phonetic description can often underestimate a disordered client's phonological ability, it can also sometimes overestimate it. This can occur when the transcribers are limited to the symbols used in a phonemic transcription of English or when they are influenced by the expected sound (or both). We show below the sample from Ball et al.'s speaker D.

Speaker D. Age 7;2. Broad transcription.

mat	[mæt͡ʂ]	pat	[pæt͡ʂ]
top	[t͡sɑːp]	tin	[t͡sɪn]
match	[mæt͡ʃ]	patch	[pæt͡ʃ]
chop	[t͡ʃɑːp]	chin	[t͡ʃɪn]

This transcription suggests that the speaker maintains a contrast between target /t/ and /tʃ/. The affricate appears to be pronounced as the adult target, with the plosive realized as an affricate at the alveolar place of articulation. However, if we examine the narrow transcription, we can see that in this instance a restriction to the symbols used in transcribing adult English have led to an overestimation of this patient's abilities:

Speaker D. Age 7;2. Narrow transcription.

mat	[mæt͡ʂ]	pat	[pæt͡ʂ]
top	[t͡ʂɑːp]	tin	[t͡ʂɪn]
match	[mæt͡ʂ]	patch	[pæt͡ʂ]
chop	[t͡ʂɑːp]	chin	[t͡ʂɪn]

This speaker uses a retroflex affricate for both target /t/ and /tʃ/. The expected alveolar and post-alveolar positions appear to have influenced the choice of symbols in the first transcription. The more detailed second transcription does demonstrate that the contrast between these phonemes is lost and will need to be re-established in therapy. Further examples of how broad transcriptions can provide misleading data are given in Carney (1979), and Ball et al. (1996) also provide a large sample of transcriptions of types of disordered speech, also showing how the extended IPA symbols for the transcription of atypical speech (extIPA, see Duckworth, Allen, Hardcastle, & Ball, 1990) are used.

However, good, accurate phonetic transcription is often difficult. There are several studies showing that the more detailed transcribers attempt to be, the more inter- and intratranscriber inaccuracies tend to occur (e.g., Shriberg & Lof, 1991). In recent times, therefore, in line with the increasing availability and simplicity of phonetic instrumentation, transcribers have more frequently integrated instrumental and impressionistic aspects of the description of both normal and disordered speech.

Ball and Rahilly (1996) describe one such example in detail. The authors were attempting a detailed impressionistic transcription of a taped sample of stuttered speech. Not only was the stutter severe, with numerous repetitions, but there were also changes in voice quality (including both breathy and creaky voice), velopharyngeal fricatives, pulmonic ingressive speech, quiet speech, and strong articulations. As well as the problem of transcribing these features, there was the added difficulty that the transcribers were working from an old tape with considerable background noise (including someone knocking on the clinic room door when the recording was made).

Nevertheless, the authors demonstrate that spectrographic analysis of the passage allowed the transcription of the whole piece with a fair degree of confidence. This kind of analysis was particularly useful during passages of very quiet repetition, with the spectrogram allowing the transcribers to calculate the number of repetitions involved at specific points. The authors note that their exercise in analysis demonstrated how useful the acoustic record can be in resolving problematic aspects of phonetic transcription. They go on to point out, however, that it must be remembered that acoustic analysis is only one instrumental technique that can be brought to bear on difficult material. Recent developments in articulatory measurement (for example, through the use of electropalatography or electrolaryngography) can help resolve transcriptional uncertainties as well; often these may be more helpful than reliance on spectrography. However, many of these techniques cannot be used with taped material, as they require the subject to be connected to the instrumentation. For a fuller examination of a range on instrumental techniques that can be used in the description of clinical speech data, see Ball and Code (1997).

REFERENCES

Ball, M. J., & Code, C. (Eds.). (1997). *Instrumental clinical phonetics*. London: Whurr.

Ball, M. J., & Rahilly, J. (1996). Acoustic analysis as an aid to the transcription of an example of disfluent speech. In M. J. Ball & M. Duckworth (Eds.), *Advances in Clinical Phonetics*. Amsterdam: John Benjamins.

Ball, M. J., Rahilly, J., & Tench, P. (1996). *The phonetic transcription of disordered speech*. San Diego: Singular Publishing Group.

Carney, E. (1979). Inappropriate abstraction in speech assessment procedures. *British Journal of Disorders of Communication, 14,* 123–135.

Duckworth, M., Allen, G., Hardcastle, W. J., & Ball, M. J. (1990). Extensions to the International Phonetic Alphabet for the transcription of atypical speech. *Clinical Linguistics and Phonetics, 4,* 273–280.

Shriberg, L., & Lof, G. (1991). Reliability studies in broad and narrow transcription. *Clinical Linguistics and Phonetics, 5,* 225–279.

CHAPTER

2

Generative Phonology

DAVID INGRAM

There are two ways in which we can define the theoretical model referred to as generative phonology. The first way is a broad definition that encompasses a wide range of theoretical assumptions concerning the nature of features, underlying and surface representations, and the mapping between representations. These assumptions were developed in the late 1950s and early 1960s and have been evolving ever since. A second, more narrow definition refers to the form in which this general theoretical orientation took in its early formulation during the 1960s. This chapter focusses primarily on the latter definition.

To appreciate the generative phonology model, it is necessary to understand the basic assumptions that underlie it and also the specific models that it has led to over the years. The earliest form of the theory dominated a range of publications in the 1960s and 1970s in linguistic theory, normal phonological acquisition, and language acquisition in children with phonological impairments. Most recently, the approach has evolved into a theoretical model often called nonlinear phonology. This approach emerged in the 1980s and is still undergoing development. It is only in the most recent years that it has been applied to phonological acquisition.

This chapter has two broad sections, the first devoted to the basic assumptions that underlie generative phonology and the second to application of the theory to phonological acquisition. The second section contains two subsections. The first subsection discusses the concept of a phonological representation in relation to normal children and children with phonological impairments. The second subsection provides a similar discussion concerning the acquisition of distinctive features. Both subsections consider the implications for treatment.

GENERATIVE PHONOLOGY: BASIC ASSUMPTIONS

Although many early articles and books can be identified as using generative phonology, the theory is most forcefully expressed in the 1968 book *The Sound Pattern of English* by Noam Chomsky and Morris Halle. The book was so influential that it became referred to by its initials SPE. SPE proposed that phonological theory consisted of two kinds of universal properties, substantive universals and formal universals. Substantive universals concern the content of phonology. The most central unit of content was and continues to be the **phonological feature**. Formal universals concern the shape of the formalism that is used to represent the substantive information. One aspect of the form of the phonology is the way that features are represented, that is, **representations**. Another is the form of the rules that operate within the phonology.

The notion that phonemes consist of phonological features had been discussed previously, such as in the work of Jakobson, Fant and Halle (1951). SPE, however, presented an explicit set of features and detailed discussion of their properties. Importantly, generative phonology rejects the notion of *phoneme*, that is, distinct sounds that distinguish the meanings of words, and proposes that the phoneme is the phonetic reflex of a small set of **distinctive features**. This can be exemplified with the English stop consonants. Phonetically, we get several variant forms, that is, voiced sounds before vowels (*bat* [bæt]), voiceless aspirated sounds before vowels (*pat* [pʰæt]), and voiceless unaspirated sounds after [s] before a vowel (*spat* [spæt]). The difference between voiced and voiceless sounds is distinctive, that is, it differentiates between two words. The phonetic feature of aspiration, however, is a predictable, or **redundant feature**. We know that a voiceless stop will be unaspirated after [s] and aspirated otherwise.

The distinction between distinctive and redundant features is important in discussing how a speaker's knowledge of their phonology is constituted. The distinctive features of a phoneme will form the **underlying representation** of that phoneme. Both the aspirated and unaspirated [p]s will be [–voice] in the underlying representations of the words in which they occur. There are also a set of **phonological rules** that operate on underlying representations to enter the predictable features. One such rule will be a rule that aspirates voiceless stops when they occur at the beginning of a syllable before a vowel and makes them unaspirated when they occur after [s]. The result of applying all the phonological rules to the underlying representations is a phonetic, or **surface representation**. The complete description of going from the underlying representation of a word through the set of phonological rules to the surface representation is called a **derivation**.

SPE discussed in great detail the nature of phonological features, the form of underlying representations, and the form of phonological rules. The establishment of a set of universal phonological features was and still is a topic of great controversy. There are a number of proposals in the literature, and linguistics textbooks differ from one another about which features are used. To the beginning student, this uncertain state of affairs can be disconcerting. The important point, however, is to be aware that researchers do not share an agreed-on set of features, and to be sure when reading any study to determine what the definitions for the features that are being used are. It is also of great importance to recognize that SPE proposed that features are binary, that is, that they have "+" or "–" values. For example, sounds are either [+voice] or [–voice] or [+aspirated] or [–aspirated].

The SPE feature system consists of several sets of features based on their acoustic and/or articulatory properties. One important set of features is the **major class features**, which, as their name indicates, mark the major classes of speech sounds. There are three major class features (note that features are commonly placed within square brackets):

- [sonorant]: sounds that can be spontaneously voiced such as vowels, nasals, liquids, and glides are [+sonorant]; other sounds (the obstruents) are [–sonorant].
- [vocalic]: sounds that have no oral constriction greater than [i] and [u] are [+vocalic], (which includes glides and liquids); otherwise they are [–vocalic].
- [consonantal]: sounds produced with a radical constriction in the oral cavity are [+consonantal] (these include obstruents, nasals, and liquids); otherwise they are [–consonantal].

These three features define at least five major classes for English as given in (1):

(1) features   major classes (with examples)

	obstruents	nasals	liquids	glides	vowels
	p,f,tʃ	m,n,ŋ	l,r	w,j,h	i,u,a
[sonorant]	–	+	+	+	+
[vocalic]	–	–	+	+	+
[consonantal]	+	+	+	–	–

Another important group of features are the **place features**, that is, the features that indicate the place in the vocal tract where sounds are produced. The more basic place features are:

- [anterior]: sounds produced at the alveolar ridge and forward are [+anterior], otherwise they are [–anterior];
- [coronal]: sounds produced with the tip or blade of the tongue are [+coronal], otherwise they are [–coronal];
- [back]: sounds produced at the soft palate are [+back], otherwise they are [–back].

We can then use these features to distinguish groups of English consonants by place, as shown in (2):

(2) features   sample consonants

	b,p,f	d,t,s	tʃ,dʒ	g,k
[anterior]	+	+	–	–
[coronal]	–	+	+	–
[back]	–	–	–	+

Used in this way, the phonological features can be used to capture explicitly the notion of **natural class**, that is, a group of sounds that share some property and undergo phonological rules as a group. Three sounds [b], [p], and [f] share the features [+anterior] [–coronal] and are part of the natural class of labials. Three other sounds such as [b], [tʃ], and [k] do not share any single set of place features and therefore do not form a natural class.

SPE also makes a number of explicit proposals about the form of phonological rules. The basic phonological rule has the form in (3):

(3) A → B / X ___ Y

This formalism is interpreted as follows: Some representation of one or more features (A) undergo a change (→ B), in some context (/ symbolizes "in the context of") of preceding sounds (X) and following sounds (Y). We can see how this formalism operates by returning to the example of English aspiration. A is the set of features that will change; in this case they need to be the features that identify the English voiceless stops. Let's assume these are at least [+consonantal], [–continuant], [–voice]. ([continuant] is the feature distinguishing stop consonants that block airflow from those that allow air to pass.) The change is that a feature is added, that is, they become [+aspirated]. The context preceding the voiceless stops is that they must be at the beginning of a syllable. Let's assume the feature [+syllable boundary] captures this. The voiceless stops must also precede a vowel, that is, a segment that is [+vocalic]. The rule then looks as:

$$(4) \qquad A \quad \rightarrow \quad B \quad / \quad X \quad \underline{} \quad Y$$

$$\begin{bmatrix} \text{+consonantal} \\ \text{–continuant} \\ \text{–voice} \end{bmatrix} \rightarrow \text{[+aspirated]} / \text{[+syllable boundary]}\underline{}\text{[+vocalic]}$$

In this example, we have added a feature. There are three other possible changes that can take place. One of these is that features can be changed. For example, in the word *smoke*, the [m] after the [s] is voiceless, that is, has assimilated to the voicelessness of the preceding consonant. The underlying /m/ which is normally [+voice] will need to be changed by a phonological rule to be [–voice]. The other two changes involve instances where entire sounds (or more accurately bundles of features) can be inserted or deleted. For example, we can pronounce a word like *play* in an exaggerated manner by inserting a brief vowel (a schwa [ə]) between the /p/ and /l/, and say [pəle]. An example of deletion is in the speech of some speakers who pronounce *can't* as [kæt]. A deletion rule is needed to delete the nasal consonant. Rules of deletion and insertion can be shown by using the symbol Ø to indicate the place where the insertion takes place or what results from the deletion. Here, (5) provides simple rules for these two examples:

(5)　a.　Insertion: Ø → [+schwa] / [+consonantal] ____ [+consonantal]

　　　b.　Deletion: [+nasal] → Ø / [+vocalic] ____ [+consonantal]

The example concerning the deletion of the nasal consonant provides an instance of another important characteristic of generative phonology.

This characteristic is referred to as **rule ordering**. When two or more phonological rules exist, they will have a fixed order in which they must be applied. In *can't* [kǽt], there is also a phonological rule that nasalizes a vowel when it is followed by a nasal consonant. This rule needs to apply before the nasal is deleted or else the context of the nasalization rule will be lost. Note that (6) shows the two possible derivations based on how these two rules are ordered. (For sake of clarity, the underlying representations are given as the phonemes /kænt/ but remember that these are just abbreviations for sets of features.)

(6) / k æ n t /   / k æ n t /

    æ̃   nasalization   Ø   nasal deletion

    Ø   nasal deletion   nasalization (cannot apply)

[k æ̃ t]   [k æ t]

The only ordering that results in the correct phonetic form is having nasalization precede nasal deletion, that is, the ordering shown on the left side of (6).

A last general aspect of the SPE approach is that it made a preliminary attempt to develop a theory of **markedness**. Markedness is the complexity of features such that some values are considered more basic (or less marked) than others. For example, it is common for sonorant consonants such as liquids and nasals to be voiced, but rare for them to be voiceless. Marking a voiced nasal as [+voice] and a voiceless one as [−voice] does not capture this. SPE suggested a way to incorporate markedness into underlying representations. The general proposal was that we could replace + and −voice values of features with "u" to indicate an unmarked value and an "m" to indicate a marked one. Before underlying representations undergo phonological rules, the u's and m's would be changed into +'s and −'s by a set of **marking conventions**. In our [voice] example, a nasal would be [u voice] with a marking convention stating that [u voice] in nasals is [+voice].

The operation of the marking conventions can be shown by applying them to the features discussed earlier. SPE suggests the markedness in (7) for any segment occurring in the initial position of a word. Vowels are considered most marked in this regard, and true consonants (the obstruents and nasals) as least marked. The liquids and glides fall in between.

(7) features   major classes (with examples)

	obstruents & nasals	liquids	glides	vowels
	p,f,tʃ,m,n,ŋ	l,r	w,j,h	i,u,a
[vocalic]	u	m	u	m
[consonantal]	u	u	m	m

An important aspect of the SPE attempt to develop formally marked and unmarked features is that it allows for quantifying markedness. This is most clearly seen in their marking conventions for vowels. (8) gives the representation for the five most basic vowels found in languages according to SPE:

(8)

features	a	i	u	e	o
[low]	u	u	u	u	m
[high]	u	u	u	m	m
[back]	u	−	+	−	−
[round]	u	u	u	u	m
[complexity]	0	1	1	2	2

Complexity is determined by adding a single point for each time either an m or a + or - (i.e., when the feature is not unmarked occurs). By these counts [a] is the least marked vowel and [e] and [o] are the most marked (of this group).

The examination of markedness proved to be a difficult matter and subsequent work has been limited. The kinds of problems can be seen in (8), where SPE needed to use + and – in some instances to make the conventions work. The difficulty of the task, however, should not blur its potential importance. Subsequent theoretical work as discussed by Dinnsen (this volume) has suggested that only marked features be represented in underlying representations. A theory along these lines leads to possible claims about acquisition, assuming that a child will acquire unmarked features before marked ones. For example, in (8) [a] is the least marked vowel so it should be predicted to be the first acquired, followed by [i] and [u], and then lastly [e] and [o].

This preliminary description of generative phonology has covered the most basic parts of the theory. The reader is encouraged to contact linguistic texts and other sources to fill in the details of the theory. This brief outline provides the foundation for the examination of how the SPE theory has been applied to the study of phonological acquisition in both normal children and children with phonological impairments. A knowledge of the theory is necessary for at least two reasons. First, it is needed to read a wide range of publications in the 1960s to 1980s in our field. Secondly, it is important to know how to understand the more current theory of nonlinear phonology. This more recent theory has evolved from the earlier one and still shares some of its most general assumptions.

GENERATIVE PHONOLOGY AND PHONOLOGICAL ACQUISITION

Representations

The major work to apply SPE generative phonology to phonological acquisition in normal children is Smith (1973). The book is a diary study of the author's son Amahl from the age of 2;2 to 3;11. It consists of phonological analyses of Amahl's phonological development and an appendix of his words. There are two major contributions of the book. First, it lays out the central implications of generative phonology for the study of phonological acquisition. Second, it provides data that has been discussed and re-analyzed ever since. A basic understanding of Smith's analyses and Amahl's data have become a prerequisite for the study of phonological acquisition.

The central theoretical theme of Smith's study concerns the *nature of the child's underlying representations*. Smith considers two options. One is that the child is capable of perceiving the adult words at an early age and constructs underlying representations that are the same as the adult surface representation of words. These underlying representations of the child are fully specified features much as we have previously discussed for the adult language. The discrepancy between the child's underlying representation and his or her phonetic forms is the result of a set of ordered phonological rules. Smith provides a detailed discussion of 25 strictly ordered rules that account for Amahl's phonetic forms. This approach more recently has come to be known as the **one-lexicon model**.

Smith's analysis of Amahl's phonology can be demonstrated by looking at his analysis of the word *zinc*. At approximately 2;4, Amahl pronounced zinc as [gɪk]. Smith proposes that three rules operate upon the underlying form: (1) a rule that deletes the nasal consonant, (2) a rule that assimilates the coronal fricative with the final velar consonant, and (3) a rule that changes the fricative into a stop. First, (9) shows this derivation using phonetic symbols that, as said earlier, represent abbreviations of features. (The symbol [ɣ] represents a voiced velar fricative)

(9) / z ɪ ŋ k /   underlying representation of *zinc*

      Ø   nasal consonant deletion

      ɣ   assimilation of coronal fricative to the velar stop

      g   change of fricative into a stop

  [gɪ k]   phonetic representation

Then, (10) provides a simplified version of the same derivation using features instead of phonetic symbols. The reader may refer to (2) for the place features involved. Also, (10) gives the number of the rule that Smith provides for each change that takes place. The only features shown are those needed for the operation of the rules. (In a more detailed presentation the underlying representations would contain a full set of features, not just those given. Also note that Smith uses the feature [syllabic] in place of [vocalic] that can be considered equivalent for the purposes of the present discussion.)

(10) /   z   ɪ   ŋ   k   /

[+coronal]	[+syllabic]	[+nasal]	[+consonantal]
[+anterior]			[−coronal]
[+continuant]			[−anterior]

                                          Ø   Rule 1

[−coronal]   Rule 19

[−anterior]

[−continuant]   Rule 24

rule 1:   [+ nasal] → Ø / [+syllabic] ___ [+consonantal]

rule 19: [+ coronal] → $\begin{bmatrix} -\text{coronal} \\ -\text{anterior} \end{bmatrix}$ / ___ [+syllabic] $\begin{bmatrix} -\text{coronal} \\ -\text{anterior} \end{bmatrix}$

rule 24: $\begin{bmatrix} + \text{continuant} \\ -\text{coronal} \end{bmatrix} \rightarrow [-\text{continuant}]$

Smith (1973) discusses an alternative to the one-lexicon model. The alternative option is to consider a child as capable of constructing a phonological representation for words that is not dependent on the adult shape of the words. Within this view, a child's underlying representation would be an **independent system**. An important aspect of this alternative is that the child's underlying representations are much closer to the phonetic form of words than in the one-lexicon model. As they contain less information, they can be considered as underspecified in relation to their form in the input language. The approach separates the child's perception of the adult form from the construction of an underlying representation. More recently this alternative has come to be called a **two-lexicon model**. This is because the child is conceived of having one set of lexical representations that deal with what the child can perceive and another set concerning what the child can produce. This distinction also captures that a young child's receptive vocabulary can be much larger than their expressive vocabulary.

We can use the *zinc* example to show how this alternative analysis operates. (11) gives an analysis first using phonetic symbols and informally stated rules. The symbol C indicates a consonant with no features for place or manner of articulation. K indicates a velar stop that is not specified for [voice].

(11) / C i K /   underlying representation of *zinc*

       K   1. an underspecified initial consonant takes on the features of a specified final consonant

      g   k   2. initial consonants are voiced, final consonants are voiceless

The child's representation in (11) contains much less information than in (9). The rules that operate are what Smith calls "morpheme structure conditions." These are statements about what can be a well-formed word. For this general discussion, however, they can be considered rules similar to those that operate in the one-lexicon model. In (12) the same derivation using features instead of phonetic symbols is shown.

(12) /   C   i   k   /

    [+consonantal]   [+syllabic]   [+consonantal]

[–syllabic]   [+high]   [–syllabic]

                    [+front]   [–continuant]

                                  [–coronal]

                                  [–anterior]

[–continuant]   Rule 1 in (11)

[–coronal]

[–anterior]

[+voice]   [–voice]   Rule 2 in (11)

Smith's conclusion was in favor of the adultlike representations (or the one-lexicon model). He gives several arguments to support his position. One argument, for example, was that Amahl was able to perceive differences between words before he was able to produce those differences such as *mouth* versus *mouse*. Another argument was that the correct formulation of the 25 phonological rules often required identification of distinctive features that were not part of Amahl's production. For example, *apple* [ɛbu] required a rule that [ə] become [u] before the lateral /l/, a consonant not found in his own articulations. Another important argument concerned the "across-the-board" nature of sound acquisition. When new sounds were acquired, they were used correctly in a range of contexts, indicating the child knew the sound perceptually.

The theoretical issue of whether children's underlying representations are adultlike or underspecified continues to be a central issue today (c.f., Menn & Matthei 1992). The reader is encouraged to consider this issue as he or she reads the other chapters in this volume. Dinnsen (Chapter 4), for example, takes a very strong position against Smith and in support of **underspecification**, a more recent term to refer to claims that children's early underlying representations are incomplete.

That researchers do not always agree on the nature of phonological representations in normal children makes the study of this topic even more difficult for children with phonological impairments. Several possible hypotheses are available. Under one view, we can claim that normal children and children with phonological impairments have more or less similar kinds of representations, whatever that might be. Phonological impairment can then be viewed as a developmental problem, that is, the development is slower. A proposal of this kind is in Ingram (1987), with the important additional observation that development in all children is highly variable, and that vocabulary acquisition needs to be considered, as well. It is suggested that the children who look the least normal are those with very reduced phonological systems and relatively large vocabularies.

A variant to this approach would be that they have similar underlying representations, but that phonologically impaired children have more problems mapping from the underlying level to the surface. This would be manifest in impaired children showing a wider range of rules and greater variability in pronunciation. Much of the research from this perspective has been done with a focus on children's **phonological processes**, that is, the phonological rules that apply between a child's underlying and surface representations. The most important work from this point of view remains Grunwell (1981), who provides detailed phonological analyses on seven children with phonological impairments. Perhaps the most striking evidence for unusual mapping is the existence of **gross inclusions** in Grunwell's data, that is, cases where several adult phonemes are reduced to a single sound. A few of the more impressive examples in the Grunwell study are shown in (13). Normal children do not commonly show such a wide range of substitutions.

(13) Child Gross Inclusion

subject 2: / f, θ s, ʃ, tʃ, dʒ, tr, dr / → [f]

/ d, g, v, ð, z, l → [v]

subject 3: / p, b, m, t, d, n, tʃ, dʒ / → [d]

subject 6: / p, t, k, g, tʃ, dʒ, f, ð, s, ʃ, l / → [t]

Still another hypothesis is to claim that normal children and children with impairments differ in their underlying representations. Under this view, phonologically impaired children are perceived as having less complete (or correct) representations than do normal children. A variant of this perspective can be found in a range of papers by Dinnsen, Gierut, and their colleagues. Dinnsen, Elbert, and Weismer (1981) propose a typology of phonologically impaired children. Two of their types capture this difference. Type A consists of children whose representations are adultlike but who may have phonological rules that obfuscate this. The data in (14a) show such a case. The child has final consonants, but deletes them at the end of a word. The evidence for the underlying consonants is the appearance of the final consonants when a final vowel is added.

> (14) a. Type A (correct underlying representations)
>
> Jamie (7;2) *cab* [kæ:], *cabby* [kæbi]
>
> *dog* [dɔ:], *doggie* [dɔgi]
>
> *duck* [dʌ], *duckie* [dʌki]
>
> Type B (incorrect underlying representations)
>
> b. Matthew (3;11) *dog* [dɔ], *red* [wɛ], *doggie* [dai], *daddy* [dæi]

At the other extreme is Type B, which represents children who have underlying representations that are very different from the adult forms. The data for Matthew in (14b) represent such a child. Matthew does not have final consonants and they do not surface even when a final vowel is added. Dinnsen et al. claim that in such cases there is no evidence for final consonants in the underlying forms of words.

A difficulty with discussing two types of children such as this is the problem of distinguishing types of children from children being at varying developmental stages. Someone defending the one-lexicon model could argue that Matthew is simply at an earlier stage than Jamie, as evidenced by his more reduced system. Smith's approach is capable of describing either type of child. Both children would have a rule that deletes postvocalic consonants. Matthew's rule is more general: It deletes any consonant that appears after a vowel. Jamie's rule is more specific: It only applies at the end of a word. (15) shows both rules using generative phonology notation.

> (15) a. Jamie: [+consonantal] → Ø / [+vocalic] _____ [+word boundary]
>
> b. Matthew: [+consonantal] → Ø / [+vocalic] _____

A related problem with determining which hypothesis is correct is that both theories are usually capable of describing the data as in the preceding example. Further, the implications for treatment of different approaches are not always apparent (c.f., Ingram, in press a). For example, Dinnsen (Chapter 4) gives the data in (16) for a child studied in Gierut (1986). This child had a phonological pattern whereby [f] occurred word initially and [s] occurred elsewhere, that is, either intervocalically or at the end of words. Although [f] and [s] are separate phonemes in adult English, they functioned as allophones in this child's phonological system:

(16)   a. [f]: *face* [fes], *food* [fu], *vine* [faɪn], *thumb* [fʌm]

     b. [s]: *wolf* [wʊsi], *goofy* [gusi], *t.v.* [tisi], *with* [wɪs]

The underspecification account proposed by Dinnsen is that fricatives do not have place features in their underlying representations and that place features are inserted by default rules. The default rules are that fricatives are [labial] if they appear in word-initial position, and [coronal] elsewhere. However, a generative phonology approach such as Smith's could propose that the child perceived the fricatives correctly, but had phonological rules that changed their place features. The implications of both accounts for treatment are the same: The child needs to produce both [f] and [s] in the same syllable positions.

It is understandable that speech-language pathologists (SLPs) can be skeptical of theoretical alternatives when it is not apparent how they lead to different treatment programs. There are, however, two reasons why it is important for SLPs to have a basic knowledge of the theoretical proposals such as those in this volume. One reason is knowledge based; the more one knows about the rationale behind a treatment model, the better one will be at assessing its strengths and weaknesses. Knowledge makes for a better consumer. The other reason is a practical one: Theoretical models have been proven to lead to better treatment methods. For example, in the previous case it is clear that treatment needs to focus on the features that underlie the distinction of [f] and [s] and the rules that result in their surface appearance. It is not a coincidence that /f/, /v/, and /θ/ become [f] word initially; they form the class of word initial fricatives.

The clinical relevance of underlying representations can also be seen in the study done by Gierut, Elbert, and Dinnsen (1987). Children with phonological impairments were divided into either Type A or Type B children as exemplified in (14) above. The Type A children were treated for the sounds that were correct underlyingly but not on the surface. For a child like Jamie, these would be the final consonants that are deleted at the end of words. Type B children were treated for those sounds that were missing in underlying representations, such as Matthew's word final consonants. The result for the Type A children was that they only improved on the treated consonants; there was not generalization to nontreated sounds. Type B children, however, showed improvements on both treated and nontreated sounds. The rationale for this effect was that the treatment led to changes in their general ability to construct underlying representations. Type A children had a less dramatic change to their systems; they only lost a rule mapping specific sounds to their surface form. No change in underlying form was involved. This is a very preliminary result, especially given that there were only three subjects in each group. It does, however, show the potential of dealing with the issue of how children represent their phonological knowledge.

Feature Acquisition

Another important contribution of generative phonology to the study of phonological acquisition is the focus on distinctive features. Earlier research such as Templin (1957) concentrated on determining the order in which particular phonemes are acquired. With the feature as the central unit in phonology, however, the focus changed to the study of the order of acquisition of distinctive features. Early efforts to do this can be found in Singh (1976) and Blache (1978). The general flavor of this work is that the unmarked or more basic features will be acquired before the more marked or less basic ones.

Although linguists agree that features constitute adult languages, there is still the central question of when children begin to acquire distinctive features. There are two basic positions on this point. One of these is the **continuity view**, which claims that children begin acquisition with the ability to represent their phonological knowledge with distinctive features. This is the original position in the first major study in phonological acquisition by the Russian linguist Roman Jakobson (Jakobson 1941/1968). It is also the position found in much recent research (e.g., Demuth & Fee, 1995; Dinnsen, 1992; Ingram, 1988; Rice & Avery, 1995). The alternative view is a **discontinuity view** found in a range of studies as well (Ferguson & Farwell, 1975; Macken, 1978; Vihman & Velleman, 1989). These researchers believe that the first words are not broken down into features, but instead are represented individually as holistic units. There is a gradual transition or shift to syllables, then to segments and finally to features as vocabulary is acquired.

When assessing this issue, it is important to place the debate within a developmental framework. The focus is on what children represent in their first 50 words or so up to around the age of 1;6. Most researchers agree that feature acquisition is being established by this point in development. Also, it is a debate that has characterized research on normal acquisition more than research on children with language impairment. The reason for this is that the latter children often have relatively advanced vocabularies in relation to their phonological systems. It is generally assumed that the phonologies of these children can be described in terms of distinctive features. Given that the focus of this chapter is on clinical phonology, we will not discuss the pros and cons of this issue. My position on this point and the one assumed in the subsequent discussion is that of continuity, as argued for in Ingram (1991, in press b). Arguments for discontinuity can be found in the works cited.

Even when we assume that children are acquiring features, there are significant difficulties in studying their acquisition. One difficulty is that phonologists have not been able to agree on the universal set of features. Related to this problem is that of determining which feature has been acquired. These two related difficulties can be seen with a very simple example. Suppose that a child has acquired the consonants /p/ and /t/. What feature has been acquired? Using SPE features, we would propose that the feature is [–coronal] with /p/ being [–coronal] and /t/ being [+coronal]. More recent feature theories, however, have replaced the feature [anterior] with the feature [labial]. Within a theory that contains both [labial] and [coronal], we then have an alternative choice. The child could be analyzed as having acquired [labial] with /p/ being [+labial] and /t/ being [–labial].

Another example of this problem is characterizing children's first nasal and oral consonants. Jakobson (1941/1968) proposed that the first consonantal opposition was between nasal and oral stops. What would this feature be? An obvious possibility is that the feature is [nasal] so that the nasal consonants are [+nasal] and the oral ones are [–nasal]. Recall, however, the discussion of the major class features in (1) and [nasal] is not a major class feature, with nasals distinguished from oral consonants by the feature [sonorant]. Using the SPE features will require the child to acquire both nasal and oral sonorant consonants (liquids) before [nasal] is acquired.

Another problem in the study of feature acquisition is that features are not always acquired across the board. For example, it is not uncommon for a child to acquire the voiced stops /b/, /d/, /g/, and then acquire the voiceless stops one by one, such as /p/, then /t/, then /k/. When the child has acquired a single minimal contrast such as /b/ versus /p/, it is certainly true that [voice] has been acquired to some degree. The child with all the complete voiced and voiceless stops, however, has a more advanced system. The acquisition of a feature requires capturing not only what is being used, but also the range of phonemes in which it occurs.

A further problem is that feature acquisition of consonants will differ depending on whether one is discussing syllable initial or syllable final position. For example, a child may have a distinction between /t/ and /s/ at the end of syllables, but change /s/ into [t] in syllable initial position. It would be misleading to say that such a child has acquired the feature [continuant] even though this is true for at least coronal consonants in syllable final position. Features commonly are acquired first in a single syllable position than spread to other ones.

Given these problems, it is not surprising that discussions concerning feature acquisition waned in the 1970s and 1980s. Most recently, however, there has been a renewed interest in feature acquisition. One line of research on feature acquisition has been research by Dinnsen et al. (1990) on 40 children they refer to as functionally misarticulating. (A good summary of this research can also be found in Dinnsen 1992.) The general methodology of their research is to establish phonetic inventories of the children's consonants and then characterize the inventory in terms of distinctive features. One such inventory is given in (17) along with a set of features for Level A, their first stage of acquisition.

(17) Level A

Features	m	n	b	d	w	j	h
[syllabic]	–	–	–	–	–	–	–
[consonantal]	+	+	+	+	–	–	–
[sonorant]	+	+	–	–	+	+	–
[coronal]	-	+	–	+	-	?	–

The feature [syllabic] is needed to distinguish consonants from vowels with [consonantal] distinguishing the glides from the true consonants. As we discussed, [sonorant] is needed for the two classes of sonorants, that is, glides versus nasals. Lastly, [coronal] distinguishes the places of articulation. (Note that there are details in the model that need some clarification such as 1. the specification for the place of [j], which needs to be [+coronal] within this system although articulatorily it is a palatal sound, and 2. the features for [h], which are not obvious.)

The next level is Level B and is distinguished by the addition of voiceless stops and velar stops. The feature [anterior] is needed to distinguish the velars and [voice] for the voice distinction. This results in the inventory in (18a), which includes the features [syllabic], [consonantal], [sonorant], [coronal], [anterior], [voice]:

(18) a. Level B Inventory   b. Basic English Inventory (Ingram 1991)

```
     m  n  ŋ          m  n
     b  d  g          b  d  g
```

```
p   t   k          p   t   k
w   j   h          f   s   h
                   w
```

There are a few comments that need to be made about this claim about early feature acquisition. One is that Levels A and B are based only on two children, so that larger numbers are needed to verify them. Second, the data are from children with phonological impairments. In (18b) is provided the basic inventory for 15 English-speaking normal children at approximately 2;0, as reported in Ingram (1991). One difference is that the Level B inventory contains [ŋ] because it is considering all syllable positions, with the (18b) inventory based only on word initial position. Second, the latter does not contain [j], because it was found to be used early but at a low rate of occurrence. Third, the basic English inventory contains the fricatives [f] and [s]. Phonologically impaired children are known to have problems particularly with fricatives, so this may be a potential difference in the order of acquisition of features between these two populations.

The other levels of feature acquisition in the Dinnsen et al. (1990) study provide an idea of how subsequent phonological development precedes in phonologically impaired children. These developments are summarized in (19):

(19)	*Levels*	*New Feature(s)*	*Potential Sounds*
	Level C	[continuant]	[f], [v], [s], [z], [ʃ]
		[delayed release]	[tʃ], [dʒ]
	Level D	[nasal]	[l] or [r]
	Level E	[strident]	[θ], [ð]
		[lateral]	both [l] and [r]

The model predicts that children will acquire at least one of the potential sounds in any level before they acquire any of the features in the subsequent levels. Subsequent research in Gierut, Simmerman, and Neumann (1994) has supported these levels, although the latter study combines Levels A and B into a single level. Gierut et al. also make predictions about the treatment of children based on these results. Dinnsen (Chapter 4) discusses these proposals.

A limitation of the study of phonetic inventories such as just discussed is that the features proposed for them are not normally based on the adult sounds that are being attempted. This is an important point since children are not creating their own phonological systems; they are discovering the system of the language that they are exposed to. If children were oriented to creating their own systems, then their underlying feature representations could be greatly different from the adult system. A simple example can suffice to demonstrate this. (14a) gives forms from a child named Jamie who produced *dog* [dɔ:] and *doggie* [dɔgi]. The analysis in Dinnsen et al. (1981) was that the child had an underlying representation of dog as /dɔg/. Other analyses, however, are available. Suppose, for example that we propose that the child had analyzed dog as /dɔk/, that is, with an underlying /k/. The analysis would require a rule that deletes a final voiceless consonant and another rule which voices the /k/ between vowels to get [dɔgi]. Such analyses are rarely suggested, but the rationale is not usually made explicit.

In Ingram (1991, p. 68), an explicit hypothesis called the **distinctive feature hypothesis** was expressed to limit the kinds of underlying representations that children may have. (20) states this hypothesis:

(20)　The distinctive feature hypothesis:

Children phonologically analyze and represent their first words in distinctive features selected from the set of available features in the words they hear.

This hypothesis would not allow the analysis of dog as /dɔk/ since the adult word does not have the feature [–voice] as part of the final consonant's features.

Returning to the issue of phonetic inventories, it is possible to demonstrate that identical phonetic inventories can have different feature systems, depending on how the child uses their sounds to represent the phonemes of the adult language. Hildegard, a normal child reported in Leopold (1947) and Matthew, a phonologically impaired child in Maxwell and Weismer (1982), both had the following simple phonetic inventory for word initial consonants: [m], [n], [b], [d], [w], [j]. This inventory (with the exception of lacking an [h]) matches the Level A inventory given in (17). The substitution patterns for the two children, however, were not the same. These are shown in (21), where square brackets indicate the child's sounds and the slashes indicate the English phonemes they represent.

(21)　a. Hildegard
　　　　[m] /m/　　　　　　[n] /n/
　　　　[b] /b,p/　　　　　 [d] /d,dʒ,t,k,g/
　　　　[w] /w,r,f/　　　　　[j] /l/

b. Matthew

[m] /m/　　　　　　　　　　[n] /n/
[b] /b,p,f,v/　　　　　　　　[d] /t,k,d,g,dʒ,tʃ,ʃ,s,θ, z/
[w] /w/　　　　　　　　　　[j] /j/

The critical differences concern [b] and [w]. For Hildegard, [b] represents labial stops and [w] replaces a glide /w/, a liquid /r/, and /f/, that is, continuants. For Matthew, [b] represents labial stops and fricatives, that is, labial obstruents, and [w] is for the glide /w/. The application of the distinctive feature hypothesis restricts the features that each child can be said to have acquired. Remember that the distinctive feature hypothesis states that the child will only assign features that are available in the input sounds. For Matthew [b] cannot be [–continuant] because it replaces the fricatives /f/, /v/ that are [+continuant]. The features that capture [b] are [–sonorant] [+labial]; [w] is [+sonorant] [+labial]. For Hildegard, however, [+sonorant] is ruled out for [w] because [w] is used for the fricative [f], which is [–sonorant]. [continuant] becomes the relevant feature: [w] is [+continuant] [+labial] and [b] is [–continuant] [+labial]. These differences are summarized in (22).

(22) Hildegard　　　　　　　　　　　　Matthew

	/b,p/	[w] /w,r,f/		[b] /b,p,f,v/	[w] /w/
[labial]	+	+	[labial]	+	+
[continuant]	–	+	[sonorant]	–	+

Differences such as these show that we need to include the English target sounds for phonetic inventories to determine accurately which features have and have not been acquired.

The differences in the two children's systems also has implications for treatment. If two children such as these were undergoing intervention, they would both need to acquire an [f]. In terms of determining a sound to be taught, the children's programs would be identical. The system that would be targeted, however, is different. Hildegard needs to acquire [sonorant], so [f] would need to be contrasted with [w]. Matthew, however, has acquired [sonorant], but needs to acquire [continuant]. [f] in his case would need to be contrasted with [b].

A last point about the features acquired at Levels A and B in Dinnsen et al. (1990) is that the child at these stages has actually acquired several sounds and features. There is no discussion of whether or not children show other stages before these levels are reached. Research on this issue is difficult because we are dealing with the earliest stage of acquisition, when children only have a few words. There is, however, one group of children who can be expected to shed light on this question.

These are the subtype of children with phonological impairments who have a severely limited phonological system, but a more advanced vocabulary.

My research on children with severely limited phonological systems indicates that children may take several different routes on their way to Levels A and B. (23) presents summaries on the word initial consonants of two children who only had acquired two consonants each.

(23) a. Kevin
        [d] /b,d,g,ð/   [t] /p,t,k/
        [+voice]   [-voice]

      b. Mike
        [n] /n,w/   [d] /d,s,ð/
        [+sonorant]   [-sonorant]

The one child, Kevin, had only acquired the distinctive feature [voice] with the other child having only acquired [sonorant]. Preliminary analyses on children with slightly more developed systems show the same kind of variability.

Data such as that presented in this section show that the determination of a child's distinctive features is a fundamental part of understanding a child's phonological system. Also, research such as that in Dinnsen et al. (1990) suggests that there is an order of acquisition to feature acquisition. The fact that a child has acquired a particular distinctive feature, however, is only part of the picture. It is also necessary to determine the extent to which the feature is used within the child's system, that is, its **functional load**. Recall the gross inclusion pattern in subject 2 in Grunwell (1981) that was given in (13) and repeated here in (24):

(24) / f, θ s, ʃ, tʃ, dʒ, tr, dr / → [f]
      / d, g, v, ð, z, l / → [v]

Subject 2 has acquired a [voice] feature which separates [f] from [v]. The [voice] feature has a large functional load in this example in that the [–voice] value for [f] is representing eight English phonemes, with the [+voice] value representing six.

The importance of examining the functional load of distinctive features can be shown by analyzing the word-initial consonants of two children. One child is John, a 6-year-old boy with a phonological impairment whose data is taken from Shriberg and Kwiatkowski (1979). The other child is my daughter Jennika at 1;7. Their phonetic inventories and the English phonemes that they are used for are in (25).

(25) a. John
      [m] /m/   [n] /n/
      [b] /b/   [d] /d, g, ð/
                    [t] /p, t, k, s/
      [w] /w, l, r/   [h] /f, h/

   b. Jennika
      [m] /n/   [n] /n/
      [b] /b, p/   [d] /d, t/   [g] /g/
      [f] /f/   [ʃ]/s, ʃ/   [Ø] /h/
      [w] /w, r, l/

There are a number of similarities between the two systems. For example, they both have two nasal consonants [n] and [m], and the voiced stops [b] and [d]. Also, both have a [w] for /w/, /l/, and /r/. The main differences are that John has no velar consonant and no fricatives except for [h], a laryngeal sound. John does, however, have one sound that Jennika doesn't, this being the voiceless stop [t].

A typical treatment program for John might include teaching the sounds that are missing from the Level A and B inventories, that is, the velars [g] and [k], the voiceless labial [p], and the glide [j]. Another alternative is to do the same using the basic English inventory in (18b). This would add the fricatives [f] and [s] to the program. Were Jennika a child to undergo therapy, there would be fewer missing sounds. The main gap would be that she has yet to acquire the voiceless stops. In terms of features, we can characterize John as lacking the feature [+back] for velars and [+continuant] for the fricatives. Jennika lacks the feature [voice].

Such analyses are descriptively correct, but they miss a central difference between John's and Jennika's system. John not only has acquired [voice], but it has an extensive functional load within his system. First, notice that the distinction between [t] /p, t, k, s/ and [d] /d, f, ð/ is being used to represent seven adult English phonemes. Also, one possible analysis of the difference between [w] /w, l, r/ and [h] /f, h/ is that it involves a [voice] difference as well, that is, [w] represents voiced continuants and [h] represents voiceless continuants. (An exception is /s/ which became [t], but some /s/ words were pronounced as [h] as well supporting this analysis.) The underlying representation of [voice] for John is given in (26).

(26) /p t k s d ð g w l r   f h / English phonemes
       [t t t t d d d w w w h h] John's consonants
[voice] −   −   −   − + + + + + +   −   −

There are at least two important points to make about such data. One is that we can't just determine whether children have or have not acquired a feature, but also need to examine the extent to which the feature is used. The second point is that this pattern is one which is typical of a subtype of children with phonological impairments, children with supralaryngeal developmental delays (Ingram 1990, in press a). We have already seen another child with this pattern, Kevin in (23a). The account for this pattern is as follows. The use of [voice] requires the use of the larynx, while distinctions such as velar [k] and fricatives involves the tongue, a supralaryngeal articulator. Children who show this pattern are having problems with supralaryngeal developments, but are capable of continuing the development of the larynx as an articulator. The result is a high functional load for [voice] at developmental stages where normal children such as Jennika may have no [voice] distinctions at all.

The identification of this pattern has important general implications for our characterization of phonological impairments as well. A typical viewpoint in the approach to children with impairments is to discuss what they lack. The feature analysis of John, however, shows that he is developing his use of [voice] at the same time that he is having difficulties with surpralaryngeal distinctions. He is developmentally delayed in terms of age, but developmentally different in terms of his phonological system. We can call this distinct development **phonological compensation**. The difficulties with surpralaryngeal articulation are compensated for by use of the larynx to capture voice contrasts.

The concept of phonological compensation may also explain another subtype of children, those with bizarre or at least highly unusual articulations (Leonard, 1985). One such case is a child who replaced word final coronal fricatives and affricates with a nasal snort (Edwards & Bernhardt, 1973). Some examples are *juice* [dɪ̃s], *brush* [bʌ̃s], and *watch* [jʌ̃s] (where [s̃] indicates the nasal snort). Another case is a child who produced an ingressive [s] (Ingram & Terselic, 1983). This is an [s] like sound made with air flowing into the oral cavity instead of out. When the [s] was prevocalic, he would also shift it to a postvocalic location. Some examples are *rouge* [wus↓], *mask* [mæs↓], *soap* [wous↓p], *spring* [wis↓] (where [s↓] indicates an ingressive [s]). While both these patterns are very unusual, they have one important effect: they allow the child to make a sound for fricatives that is distinct from other sounds in their systems. That is, the underlying feature [continuant] is reflected in some way in their speech. Such data show that these children are capable of acquiring phonological systems and actively seek means to compensate for their difficulties.

CONCLUSION

Generative phonology was a paradigm shift in phonological theory of enormous impact. Its effect on both normal phonological acquisition and phonological disorders in children was and continues to be a major influence. This chapter has concentrated on two major themes in generative phonology: 1. the abstract nature of phonological representations, and 2. the role of the distinctive feature as the basic unit of phonological organization.

The chapter began with a discussion of the basic assumptions of generative phonology. The basic structure of phonological knowledge consists of an abstract underlying representation of phonological features and a set of strictly ordered phonological rules that map from the underlying representation to the phonetic representation. Chomsky and Halle's *The Sound Pattern of English* (SPE) proposed explicit claims about these basic components. The underlying structure of phonemes are sets of distinctive features that are binary, that is, they have + and – values. The features are not ordered within their bundles, but they do consist of subgroups of features that differ in their generality. The most general features are the major class features, which determine the major classes of speech sounds (e.g. obstruents, nasals, glides, liquids and vowels). Other groupings consist of features for place and manner. Rules within the SPE model have specific formal properties concerning how they refer to sets of features and alter them. Finally, SPE also offered some initial suggestions on how to capture the markedness of features in terms of marking conventions.

The notion of underlying representation has been a central issue in the study of phonological acquisition. Smith (1973) was a major work exploring how children may represent their phonological knowledge in the early period of development. Using diary data from his son Amahl, Smith gave detailed analyses of Amahl's phonology within the SPE model. He compared one analysis that assumed that Amahl's underlying knowledge was complete in relation to adult phonetic structures, with an alternative in which Amahl had an independent (and incomplete) system of phonological representations. Smith's conclusions were in support of the former model that today is often referred to as a one-lexicon model. Both these analytic approaches have been used in the discussion of the phonological knowledge of children with phonological impairments. One line of research has taken Smith's model and analyzes impaired children with a focus on the rules (or phonological processes) that map from well-formed underlying representations to phonetic representations (e.g., Grunwell, 1981). Other work has proposed that these children have incomplete representations, and that treatment needs to focus on the establishment of underlying knowledge, not just the mapping rules (Gierut et al., 1987).

Feature acquisition has also been a central theme in research on normal children and children with impairments. Dinnsen (1992) has proposed five levels of feature acquisition based on detailed analyses of misarticulating children. The establishment of an orderly sequence of feature acquisition can be used to determine what features to teach children. Additional research is needed to determine more on the earliest stages of feature development. Preliminary results indicate that there is a statistical tendency for certain features to be acquired before others, but that individual children may vary greatly in their precise orders. The determination of a specific child's features also requires the consideration of a child's patterns of substitution. Two children with the same phonetic inventories may nonetheless have different feature systems. The study of features versus phonemes also has led to the identification of a subtype of children with phonological impairments who acquire the feature [voice] relatively early when compared to normal children of comparable phonological development. Such data indicate that these children are active learners who compensate for difficulties with supralaryngeal properties by continuing to acquire the [voice] feature that involves the larynx. The idea that children with phonological impairments compensate may also account for some of the more unusual patterns found in case studies.

Many specific formal devices and features in generative phonology have fallen out of practice within phonological theory. It is important to recognize, however, that its central tenets remain. The present article has attempted to demonstrate this point concerning representations and features. These insights have led to considerable gains in our understanding of phonological acquisition, and will continue to do so in the years ahead.

REFERENCES

Blache, S. (1978). *The acquisition of distinctive features*. Baltimore: University Park Press.

Chomsky, N., & Halle, M. (1968). *The sound pattern of English*. New York: Harper & Row.

Demuth, K., & Fee, J. (1995). *Minimal words in early phonological development*. Unpublished manuscript, Brown University and Dalhousie University.

Dinnsen, D. (1992). Variation in developing and fully developed phonetic inventories. In C. A. Ferguson, L. Menn, & C. Stoel-Gammon (Eds.), *Phonological development: models, research, implications* (pp. 191–210), Timonium, Md.: York Press.

Dinnsen, D., Chin, S.B., Elbert, M., & Powell, T. W. (1990). Some constraints on functionally disordered phonologies: Phonetic inventories and phonotactics. *Journal of Speech and Hearing Research, 33,* 28–37.

Dinnsen, D., Elbert, M., & Weismer, G. (1981). Some typological properties of functional misarticulation systems. In W. O. Dressler (Ed.), *Phonologica 1980.* (pp. 83–88) Innsbruck: Innsbruck Beiträge zur Sprachwissenschaft.

Edwards, M. L., & Bernhardt, B. (1973). *Phonological analyses of the speech of four children with phonological disorders.* Unpublished manuscript, Stanford University.

Ferguson, C. A., & Farwell, C. (1975). Words and sounds in early language acquisition: English initial consonants in the first fifty words. *Language, 51,* 419–439.

Gierut, J. (1986). Sound change: A phonemic split in a misarticulating child. *Applied Psycholinguistics, 7,* 57–68.

Gierut, J., Elbert, M., & Dinnsen, D. (1987). A functional analysis of phonological knowledge and generalization learning in misarticulating children. *Journal of Speech and Hearing Research, 30,* 462–479.

Gierut, J., Simmerman, C., & Neumann, H. (1994). Phonemic structures of delayed phonological systems. *Journal of Child Language, 21,* 291–315.

Grunwell, P. (1981). *The nature of phonological disability in children.* New York: Academic Press.

Ingram, D. (1987). Categories of phonological disorder. *First international symposium on specific language impairment in children* (pp. 88–99). Middlesex, England: Association for All Speech Impaired Children.

Ingram, D. (1988). Jakobson revisited: Some evidence from the acquisition of Polish. *Lingua, 75,* 55–82.

Ingram, D. (1991). Toward a theory of phonological acquisition. In J. Miller (Ed.), *Research perspectives on language disorders.* Boston: College–Hill Press.

Ingram, D. (in press a). The categorization of phonological impairment. In B. Hodson & M. L. Edwards (Eds.) *Applied phonology pioneers: Theoretical perspectives and clinical implications.* Frederick, MD: Aspen.

Ingram, D. (in press b). Phonological acquisition. In M. Barrett (Ed.), *The development of language.* London: UCP Press.

Ingram, D., & Terselic, B. (1983). Final ingression: A case of deviant child phonology. *Topics in Language Disorders, 3,* 45–50.

Jakobson, R. (1941/1968). *Child language, aphasia, and language universals* (A.R. Keiler, trans.) The Hague: Mouton. (Original work published 1941)

Jakobson, R., Fant, G., & Halle, M. (1951). *Preliminaries to speech analysis.* Cambridge, MA: MIT Press.

Leonard, L. (1985). Unusual and subtle phonological behavior in the speech of phonologically disordered children. *Journal of Speech and Hearing Research, 24,* 389–405.

Leopold, W. (1947). *Speech development of a bilingual child: A linguist's record. Vol. 2: Sound learning in the first two years.* Evanston, IL: Northwestern University Press.

Macken, M. (1978). Developmental reorganization of phonology: a hierarchy of basic units of acquisition. *Lingua, 49*, 11–49.

Maxwell, E., & Weismer, G. (1982). The contribution of phonological, acoustic, and perceptual techniques to the characterization of a misarticulating child's voice contrast for stops. *Applied Psycholinguistics, 3*, 29–43.

Menn, L., & Matthei, E. (1992). The "two-lexicon" account of child phonology: Looking back, looking forward. In C. A. Ferguson, L. Menn, & C. Stoel-Gammon (Eds.), *Phonological development: Models, research, implications* (pp. 211–247). Timonium, MD: York Press.

Rice, K., & Avery, P. (1995). Variability in a deterministic model of language acquisition: A theory of segmental elaboration. In J. Archibald (Ed.), *Phonological acquisition and phonological theory* (pp. 63–79). Hillsdale, NJ: Lawrence Erlbaum Associates.

Shriberg, L., & Kwiatkowski, J. (1979). *Natural process analysis (NPA)*. Madison: University of Wisconsin.

Singh, S. (1976). *Distinctive features: Theory and validation*. Baltimore: University Park Press.

Smith, N. (1973). *The acquisition of phonology: A case study*. Cambridge, England: Cambridge University Press.

Templin, M. (1957). Certain language skills in children. *University of Minnesota Institute of Child Welfare Monograph Series 26*. Minneapolis: University of Minnesota Press.

Vihman, M., & Velleman, S. (1989). Phonological reorganization: A case study. *Language and Speech, 32*, 149–170.

CHAPTER

Natural Phonology

PAMELA GRUNWELL

Natural phonology rose rapidly to a position of pre-eminence in Clinical Phonology at the end of the 1970s and early 1980s. This was largely due to the works of Hodson (1980), Ingram (1976, 1981), Shriberg and Kwiatkowski (1980), and Weiner (1979). These clinical assessment procedures, however, are based on highly simplified frameworks of analysis, which, for the most part, ignore the complex issues addressed by the theory from which they are derived.

Chronologically, natural phonology followed generative phonology into clinical phonology and has enjoyed much greater success. There are several reasons for this, which are enumerated at the beginning of this chapter as signposts to the clinical applications of this theoretical model. This is necessary because the theoretical exposition of natural phonology is based on the publications of its proponent, Stampe (1969, 1979) and with his co-author Donegan, in Donegan and Stampe (1979), who make no reference to the possible clinical relevance of the theory.

First, natural phonology has none of the formalism and quasimathematical formulae required to write phonological rules in the generative model. Second, the basic concept of natural phonology—the phonological process–can be defined relatively simply and as such is easily related to many of the descriptions of atypical speech provided in the traditional error analysis framework. Finally, as a theory natural phonology is attractive because it uses data from child phonologies and phonological development as major evidence in support of its premises.

The theory of natural phonology, as proposed by its originator, Stampe, was not and is not related to current or new approaches to phonological theory, especially generative phonology. This was well recognized by exponents of the latter theory. In his introduction to *Current Approaches to Phonological Theory*, Dinnsen (1979) concludes that the majority of approaches described in the volume are not fundamentally different; they are all versions of post-standard generative theory, "with the possible exception of Natural phonology" (p. xii). This is a viewpoint echoed by McCawley (1979) in the same volume; he regards Donegan and Stampe's (1979) chapter as an exposition of "a really comprehensive theory of phonology" (p. 294). Householder (1979) also confirms this conclusion from a somewhat different perspective. He suggests that with reference to the axioms of generative phonology, natural phonology "rejects the whole enterprise" (p. 260). He concludes that natural phonology does not subscribe to the aims of generative linguistics (Chapter 2). He states that its contribution is to "the theory of language acquisition and of phonological performance" (p. 260).

In fact, in their chapter in Dinnsen's collection, Donegan and Stampe (1979) clearly identify that natural phonology is different: it ". . . is a modern development of the oldest explanatory theory of phonology" (p. 126). The sources of this *new* phonology are the founders of phonology, who sought to establish links between diachronic phonetics, dialectal variations, synchronic variations, and child speech, (among others, Donegan & Stampe cite Sweet, 1877; Passy, 1890; Grammont, 1933; Jespersen, 1964). These discerning linguistic phoneticians sought to establish a natural explanation or causation for the phenomena they describe. The phonologists who continued this tradition, according to Stampe and Donegan (1979), are Sapir (1921, 1933) and Jakobson (1941/1968), who addressed the issues of the reality of phonological analysis and of universal phonologies in the context of the *phonetic bases* of human language. Contrary to generative theory, Donegan & Stampe (1979) argue that it is not helpful to propose that the universal characteristics of language are innate: this is not an explanation of language universals; it begs the question why? In regard to phonology, this question can be answered by looking for phonetic explanations; this is the theoretical basis of natural phonology.

THE THEORY OF NATURAL PHONOLOGY

The definitive exposition of the theory of natural phonology is presented by Donegan and Stampe (1979). Their basic premise is that the living sound patterns of language, in their development by individuals and in their evolution over the centuries of language change, are governed by natural forces in human systems of vocalization and auditory perception. It is argued that the phonological dimension of language is a natural reflection of the needs, capacities and world of its users. Explanations in natural phonology therefore focus on the fact that *language is spoken*. This is reflected in the data that are used as evidence in support of the theory. These include diachronic studies of phonological change, children's speech and speech development, comparisons between formal and casual speech, the characteristics of English "slips of the tongue," and of secret languages based on English, such as Pig Latin.

The first published statement of theory of natural phonology is Stampe's (1969) paper entitled *"The Acquisition of Phonetic Representation,"* which employs evidence from child speech as its primary database. This paper defines the theoretical framework, and although there are appreciable changes in subsequent statements with regard to the details of the analytical exposition, the fundamental concepts remain unchanged in Stampe (1979) and Stampe and Donegan (1979). According to Stampe (1969), the theory of natural phonology is "based on the assumption that the phonological system of a language is largely the residue of an innate system of phonological processes, revised in certain ways by linguistic experience." (Stampe, 1979, p. vii).

Phonological Process

The key to the theory is the concept of "phonological process," a phenomenon which is both innate and natural. Stampe provides definitions for this concept in his 1969 paper and his dissertation published in 1979. These are: "A phonological process merges a potential phonological opposition into that member of the opposition which least tries the restrictions of the human speech capacity" (1969; see 1979, p. vii).

"A phonological process is a mental operation that applies in speech to substitute, for a class of sounds or sound sequences presenting a common difficulty to the speech capacity of the individual, an alternative class identical but lacking in the difficult property" (1979, p. 1). This concept underlies the theory of natural phonology.

The premise of these definitions is that the speech mechanisms of both children and adults determine the nature of phonological systems. Stampe argues, especially in his first paper, that the characteristics of child speech are determined by the physiological constraints of the speech mechanism, "in its language-innocent state, the innate phonological system expresses the full system of restrictions of speech" (1969; see 1979, p. ix). Given this perspective, it is clear why child speech data are such an important source of evidence for the theory of natural phonology.

To illustrate the key concepts introduced thus far, an example used in all three publications by Stampe is apposite. Physiologically, voiced obstruents, especially plosives, are more difficult to produce than voiceless obstruents, because the simultaneous oral and velic closures obstruct the continuous air flow that is necessary to sustain vocal fold vibrations that produce voicing. Therefore, it is natural for obstruents to be voiceless; this is a pattern that has been observed in child speech. However, as Stampe is quick to point out, no speech sound segment occurs in isolation. Contextual factors may account for a contradictory natural process such that obstruents are voiced when they are in a voiced environment, especially when surrounded or followed by naturally voiced segments such as vowels. This illustration defines the natural phonological process of context sensitive voicing, (discussed later). Stampe, however, never uses this terminology, which is only found in the publications of interpreters of the theory, describing its potential applications in the clinical context.

The Phonetic Base of Natural Phonology

Stampe is concerned with exploring the nature of *real* human speech. He quite explicitly states that he addresses issues fundamental to the scientific investigation of language. In his thesis, he unequivocally rejected the then prevailing ethos in structuralist and generative phonology. This is especially evident in his rejection of the competence/performance dichotomy. It is clear that this concept is alien to the conceptual basis of natural phonology: "There has been a tendency in linguistics to view processes of grammar as descriptions of the language 'competence' of speakers, and not of the actual processes that occur in the production or perception ('performance') of speech" (1979, p. 43). Natural phonology, on the contrary, is clearly rooted in a phonetic base. Stampe emphasizes that the performance/competence distinction is implausible because, "it becomes increasingly clear that in general the conditions of the *use* of language (performance) are responsible for the *nature* of language. This is not by any means a peculiarity of phonology, but phonology presents a particularly striking case" (Stampe, 1979, p. 43).

The essence of phonology and of speech is therefore physical in teleology. In other words, "Although phonological substitution is a mental operation, it is clearly motivated by the physical character of speech—its neurophysiological, morphological, mechanical, temporal, and acoustic properties" (Stampe, 1979, p. 6).

It is evident from this discussion that natural phonology potentially had its own agenda: refining the concept of phonological process and identifying such processes, providing evidence of the universality of these natural processes, and cataloging and justifying a definitive set of universal processes. In fact, natural phonology had its agenda subverted by the preoccupations of the other concurrent phonological theory: generative phonology. This is clearly evident in Stampe's thesis (1979) and the chapter by Stampe and Donegan (1979) in a volume dominated by generative phonologists. With the perspective of time and the recognition that all theories are inadequate and incomplete, it is unfortunate for natural phonology that its concerns were diverted from the exploration of the physical nature of phonology to matters of formalism such as rule-ordering.

Indeed, Donegan and Stampe, even in the alien context of Dinnsen's volume on contemporary issues in generative phonology, raise issues that identify the basic tensions in *real speech*: the need for clarity in the delivery of the message in competition with ease in the effort to produce the signals that embody the message. Naturalness therefore explains the difference between the more formal styles of speech where clarity is sought through *fortition*, that is intensification of salient features of segments that render them perceptibly more different, by comparison with more casual styles of speech where ease of effort is achieved by *lenition*, where the articulatory distance between segments is decreased largely through the interaction of context sensitive factors. For example:

(1) Formal ['ɑnt ju mɪs 'dʒeɪn] and casual ['ɑntʃʊ mɪʃ 'dʒeɪn] for *aren't you Miss Jane.*

Natural phonology as a theory is potentially directly relevant to the clinical context, as it is clearly addressing real speech. In its clinical applications, however, these fundamental issues are bypassed in representations of the theory that are simplistic. Before considering these applications, those theoretical statements in the original exposition of the theory that are relevant to subsequent clinical applications are examined.

Natural phonology provides a cogent definition of the concept of natural classes: they are literally *a matter of fact*, not the products of a linguistic formalism that requires phonological rules to conform to a simplicity formula. Natural classes are defined by the physical realities of speech. One of the examples Donegan and Stampe (1979) suggest is the occurrence of nasalization of vowels and other nonnasal sonorants in English. Nasalization only occurs in the context of nasals; it is a natural process that reduces effort whilst not impairing efficiency, because it naturally only occurs on classes of sounds that are not jeopardized by nasalization, that is, sonorants (vowels and approximants), thus for example:

(2) *can; name; film* [kãn; nẽɪm; fɪ̃lm].

This introduces the issue of the range of phonological processes. Each phonological process applies to a natural class "sharing a common articulatory, perceptual, or prosodic difficulty to a common degree" (Donegan & Stampe, 1979, p. 137). Furthermore, a phonological process only changes one phonetic property or feature to overcome a phonetic difficulty: in other words "a process normally changes only one feature" (Donegan & Stampe 1979, p. 137). It is quite clearly stated that "telescoping" of processes is impossible because each process has an identifiable natural causality that needs to be identified to explain the natural processes that underlie any specific pronunciations.

Processes, Rules, and Ordering

This immediately evokes the question that is hotly debated in formalized phonologies: Is there ordering of rules/processes? In his original exposition of the theory in his dissertation, Stampe (1979, pp. 63–69) argues that, "processes naturally apply in sequence" (p. 63). In a footnote addressing this issue and in the chapter by Donegan and Stampe (1979), a different, albeit interim, position is indicated—that all processes apply simultaneously. The implication of this later hypothesis is that whatever natural processes can potentially apply, will apply and are not ordered.

The issue of ordering leads Stampe on to the issue of processes versus rules. He argues (1979, p. 47) that the distinction between processes and rules represents a fundamental difference: processes are (innate) "constraints which the speaker brings to the language" and rules are "the constraints the language brings to the speaker" (p. 47). In support of this distinction, Stampe cites the natural phonological *process* of palatalization evident in English casual/conversational speech when apical /t/ or /d/ precede palatal /j/, such as *what you* [wɒtʃʊ] or *did you* [dɪdʒʊ] in contrast to the morphophonological alternation *rule* exemplified in *electric/electricity* where /k/ → /s/. Stampe suggest that the facetious pronunciation *electrickity* demonstrates that there is no fundamental articulatory difficulty in the sequence /kɪ/, whereas articulatory effort (or fortition) is required to resist /tj/ → [tʃ].

In dealing with the issues of ordering and of rules versus processes, the published presentations of the theory of natural phonology (Stampe, 1979; Donegan & Stampe, 1979) confront the minutiae of examples of phonological change in diachronic and synchronic phonologies. These issues are not relevant to the concerns of this chapter.

The Acquisition of Phonology

However, these detailed explorations contrast markedly with the theoretical approach to the acquisition of phonology in childhood. Stampe contends that learning to pronounce involves suppressing or limiting the innate phonological system so that the child's pronunciations move closer to the adult target system. Stampe suggests (1969; see 1979 pp. xi–xii) that attributing the regularities of phonological acquisition to natural phonological processes obviates the need for "implicational laws" as proposed by Jakobson (1941). Stampe cites Jakobson's contention that no phonological system includes affricates unless it also contains plosives and fricatives. Stampe suggests that two context-free natural processes account for this: stops (i.e., plosives) are the first most natural obstruents and therefore the first natural substitution for both affricates and fricatives (or "spirants," Stampe's term). When fricatives begin to develop, they are then natural phonological substitutions for affricates. This explanation is subtly different from Jakobson's in that Stampe invokes the notion that these phenomena are attributable to naturally determined laws in the phonetic sense, rather than the structuralist viewpoint that, according to Stampe, Jakobson adopts.

Stampe also assumes a clear position with regard to the nature of a child's knowledge of the target phonological system. He asserts (1969; see 1979, p. xiii) that there is no evidence to support the view that a child has his or her own phonemic system, going on to suggest that a child's underlying representations are close to—that is, essentially the same as—adult pronunciations. He recognizes that this claim is crucial to establishing the validity of his theory that a child's pronunciations result from the application of innate phonological processes to an underlying phonological representation of individual words. Stampe (1969; see 1979, pp. xiii–xiv) and Donegan and Stampe (1979, p. 169) justify this proposal by citing evidence that children make spontaneous "across-the-board" changes on learning to pronounce accurately a new contrastive segment that had previously been merged. It is noteworthy that Smith (1973), using a generative phonological approach (Chapter 2), advances the same argument. Thus Stampe, like Smith, asserts that a child who has previously pronounced target /k/ as [t], will, on having mastered [k], only use the new consonant in those contexts and words where it is appropriate. Any instances of apparent over-generalization can be attributed, according to Stampe, to other natural context-sensitive processes such as might occur in, for example, *cat* [kak] and *dog* [gɒg], which is consonant harmony.

Stampe's view of phonological development, as Kiparsky and Menn (1977) observe, is essentially a deterministic one in that a child knows the phonological representation of the target and has to, in some way, adjust or suppress the natural tendencies of the speech-producing mechanism to achieve an accurate representation of that target. Although Stampe identifies naturalness as attributable to the auditory as well as physiological dimensions of the speech production mechanism, there is a strong implication that the major factors are articulatory.

Finally, if phonological processes are innate and therefore universal, phonological development should follow a very similar progression the world over. Stampe, however, illustrates how individual children evidence the processes in idiosyncratic ways. He discusses in particular the child pronunciation of *lamb* as [zab] and [jæ˞], focusing on the apparently very different realisations of /l/ (Stampe 1979, pp. 11–12). His analysis states that in both realizations, [l] is delateralized to [j] a common child realization for this target that is also found in diachronic sound change, such as Italian *bianco*, compared with French *blanc*. The [j] realization is then fricated to [ʒ], a change also evidenced diachronically in the change of Latin [j] in *Julius* to [ʒ] in French: *Jules* and to [dʒ] in Italian: *Giulio*. The [ʒ] is then depalatalized to [z], a common process evidenced in the realizations of many children's attempts at target palatoalveolars such that /ʃ/ becomes [s] in English: *shoe* [su] and French *chambre* [sãbr]. By this example, Stampe demonstrates that an apparently unusual child realization /l/ → [z] can be accounted for by identifying a number of interacting processes that can be found in both child speech and diachronic sound change. Furthermore, they can be said to be natural.

Summary

To conclude this theoretical overview of natural phonology, it is important to highlight the points of the theory as expounded by Stampe that have potential clinical relevance. In natural phonology, explanations of the characteristics of spoken language are based on the phonetic nature of speech. It would appear that Stampe primarily concentrates on articulatory factors; nonetheless, he does include acoustic properties in his list of the physical characteristics of speech. This then is a theory dealing with "real speech," or performance data, not the abstract underlying morphophonological representations of generative phonology. Secondly, the phonetic substrate of spoken language is manifested by natural phonological processes, which are the basic analytical concepts of the theory. Whilst these processes are not only natural but also innate, Stampe never suggests that they occur inflexibly and deterministically.

Indeed, his example of the different child pronunciations of *lamb* is used to demonstrate how children (and languages) reach different naturally motivated solutions to the constraints of spoken language. He emphasizes how processes can *co-occur* in different combinations, thus resulting in individual pronunciations of the same word. Finally, the existence and importance of natural classes are the inevitable teleological consequence of the concept of natural phonological processes.

CLINICAL APPLICATIONS

As has already been indicated, the basic analytical concept of natural phonology is eminently applicable in clinical assessment, diagnosis, and treatment. Stampe, himself, in a statement quoted previously (1979, p. 6) refers to **the phonological process** as a "phonological substitution." When the concept of phonological process became more widely known in the clinical field after the publication of Ingram's (1976) *Phonological Disability in Children*, several readily comparable sets of natural phonological processes were published as clinical assessment procedures for child speech. These included several processes not mentioned as such by Stampe; for example velar fronting and final consonant deletion, although Stampe does give examples of both (1969; see 1979, p. xiv); and processes not discussed at all by Stampe, for example the patterns of initial cluster reduction in child speech. These processes are defined and discussed in the next few pages. The question here is: Do these clinical procedures and their sets of processes represent an application or an extension of the theory? These newly defined processes describe data observed in child speech; they are therefore further evidence in support of the theory. Furthermore, the clinical assessment procedures using phonological processes are essentially descriptive frameworks (the position adopted clearly by Stoel-Gammon & Dunn, 1985, p. 113; and somewhat equivocally by Grunwell, 1985, p. 53).

As discussed later, the theoretical implications of applying natural phonology in the clinical context are addressed in several instances. In addition there are some clinical applications of the conceptual framework that address theoretical and applied theoretical concerns through an exploration of diagnostic and explanatory issues. It is, indeed, surprising that clinical data were not and have not been used in the development of the theory of natural phonology, as what one might term "unnatural conditions" provide a different perspective on what is natural. Nonetheless, the explanatory basis of natural phonology is readily accessible clinically. This is indicated in a paper that, surprisingly, makes no reference to this theory:

> The naturalness of particular phonological phenomena . . . has to do with the extent to which their occurrence can be accounted for by reference to external factors whose domain is the natural world rather than language itself. In connection with phonology, the relevant external factors are generally supposed to derive from such areas as articulatory physiology, acoustic phonetics, or perceptual psychology. It is thus perfectly possible for a child's speech to exhibit phonological patterns which are deviant [from the developmental norm, P.G.] but which are nonetheless natural to the extent that they are attributable to external phenomena of this type. (Harrris & Cottam, 1985, pp. 73–74)

This quotation suggests that there is the potential to develop a theory of natural clinical phonology. It is quite possible that this theory in essence exists, but it is not within the context of the linguistic theory of natural phonology. It is in the applied multidisciplinary context of speech and language pathology and therapy where linguistic and phonetic approaches are refracted through anatomical, physiological, neurological, and pathological lenses.

Assessment: Application in Descriptive Clinical Frameworks

It is interesting to examine how natural phonology entered significantly into the clinical context. It was through the publication of Ingram's (1976)

Phonological Disability in Children. (There was one earlier unpublished paper: Edwards & Bernhardt, 1973, which Ingram refers to.) Ingram, somewhat misleading, relates Stampe's theory to generative phonology, but compares Stampe's account of children's speech to Jakobson (Ingram, 1976, p. 4). He uses the approaches of both Stampe and Jakobson in his analysis of child phonology in his Chapter 2, and effectively swings the balance in favor of phonological processes halfway through that chapter, which forms the basis for the clinical assessment procedures that have been subsequently devised.

These assessment procedures were developed directly out of the approach taken by Ingram, which is summarized as: [from] "1;6 to 4;0 when many words are incorrectly pronounced, there are several very general simplifying processes that affect entire classes of sounds" (Ingram, 1976, p. 29).

It is clear that Ingram is trying to establish an approach to speech development that not only embraces the phonological dimension of learning the patterns of pronunciation, but also identifies that developmental changes in pronunciation affect natural classes of target sounds, thus resulting in patterns of what might be called "mispronunciations." He goes on to examine how this analytical approach may be used to investigate the deviant pronunciation development of one individual and in a later chapter how it explains the characteristics of different pronunciation disorders.

If Ingram introduced the ideas of natural phonology to the clinical context, then Weiner confirmed their relevance in 1979 when he stated that Ingram had "recommended that a speech-sampling procedure be designed that is compatible with analysis by phonological process. It is to this end that PPA (Phonological Process Analysis) was developed" (Weiner, 1979, p. 1). Hodson in 1980 is apparently less dependent on Ingram and draws on generative phonological sources such as Oller (1973) and Smith (1973), while couching the assessment framework entirely in terms of phonological processes or patterns that are found in the speech of children with severe phonological disorders as well as normal phonological development. Shriberg and Kwiatkowski (1980), on the other hand, concentrate on describing a clinical assessment procedure that reflects Ingram's suggestions about the clinical applications of natural phonology with some references back to the origins of the theory (see more discussion later). But, Ingram (1981), himself, retains a strictly descriptive approach to the concept of phonological process. This is also the approach taken by Grunwell (1985) and by Howell and Dean (1991, p. 19; original reference: Dean, Howell, Hill, & Waters, 1990), following Grunwell (1985, 1987). Stampe's theoretical definition of phonological process has been quoted in an earlier section of this chapter. It is important to examine the applied definitions of this fundamental concept. Ingram's (1976) general definition has already been quoted (see previous). Weiner (1979) similarly seeks to emphasize the presence of patterns in children's apparently individual mispronunciations: "These phonological processes are predictions of how and why the child's speech is produced as it is. Generally, the phonological processes are based on such factors as sound environment, syllable structure and use of feature contrasts" (p. 1). On the basis of this definition, Weiner seeks to relate all the processes he describes to what he ascribes to be natural factors. Weiner (1984) takes a more reflective approach to the application of phonological theory, as discussed in more detail later.

Hodson (1980) surprisingly provides no overall definition of phonological process; however, it is evident from a statement in her preface that she is employing the concept as a descriptive tool: "Recent phonological research has identified systematic patterns which may be targeted across phonemes" (p. i). In a later publication (Hodson, 1982), more definitive general statements are made in that phonological processes provide ". . . new alternatives for analyzing and categorizing articulatory deviations" (Hodson, 1982, p. 97). Also, a definition is provided in a footnote:

> The term "phonological process" is used here to simply describe a change which affects a whole class of sounds. For example, the final consonants may be deleted (*bed* → /bɛ/) or clusters may be reduced (*spoon* → /pun/). The primary concern at this time has been to identify priority patterns that can be expeditiously remediated. (Hodson, 1982, p. 99)

The whole of the footnote is quoted here as it indicates the primary focus of Hodson's use of phonological process analysis: to determine treatment priorities; this is discussed further.

Shriberg and Kwiatkowski (1980; see also Shriberg, 1982) adopt a much more complex stance on the nature of phonological processes drawing mainly, but not only, on the theoretical views as directly expressed by Stampe (reference is also made to the perceptual and physiological investigations of Locke, subsequently expressed in full theoretically in 1983b). Notwithstanding a preliminary exploration of the theoretical implications of the basic concept and the list of 43 potential natural processes in child phonology, Shriberg and Kwiatkowski (1980, p. 5) choose to limit severely the scope of their natural phonological analysis procedure. They propose eight processes (or "putatively 'natural' sound changes" Shriberg 1982, p. 45) that fulfill the following criteria:

1. They result in the simplification of speech production and are widely attested in natural language data (i.e., they have "face validity" [Shriberg, 1982, p. 45]).
2. They involve phoneme deletions and/or phoneme substitutions (which simplify phonological forms) not lower level distortions that "reflect articulatory imprecision" (Shriberg & Kwiatkowski, 1980, p. 10).
3. They occur frequently in the speech of children with delayed language development (see Shriberg, 1982, p. 45 for a clear statement of this criterion).
4. Their transcription reliability has been established (to the satisfaction of the authors) for the outcomes of the processes.

In effect, these natural processes are defined empirically and pragmatically; their theoretical status is tenuous.

Ingram (1981) provides definitions that are superficially descriptive: "Phonological processes refer to kinds of changes, which apply to classes of sounds, not just individual sounds, that children make in simplifying adult speech" (Ingram, 1981, p. 6). This is restated later as: "a simplifying tendency on the part of the child to alter natural classes of sounds in a systematic way" (Ingram, 1981, p. 77). However, Ingram indicates that he regards phonological process analysis as more than a description: "an attempt to explain a child's substitutions by describing them in terms of general patterns of simplification" (Ingram, 1981, p. 77).

Grunwell (1985) also refers to the potential explanatory value of process analysis: "The processes describe the relationship between the patterns in the adult and child pronunciations. Theoretically, this description is given explanatory power in that the processes are said to encapsulate a tendency towards *simplification* in children's speech" (p. 53). Grunwell, however, is sceptical of this explanatory power, (see further later and Locke, 1983 (a)).

It is evident from these various definitions that the concept of phonological process in the clinical assessment of child speech is applied primarily as a descriptive device that identifies or analyzes systematic patterns in children's pronunciations by comparison with the target adult pronunciations. The notion that as a consequence of the process(es) children's patterns are simpler is also a consistent factor in the definition of the concept.

Classification of Phonological Processes in Child Speech

Each of the clinical assessment procedures referred to in the preceding section classifies phonological processes differently. Table 3–1 lists the

Table 3–1. Clinical Assessment Procedures Using Phonological Process Analysis.

Weiner (1979)	Shriberg & Kwiatkowski (1980)	Hodson (1980)
Syllable Structure Process	1. Final Consonant	*Basic Phonological Processes*
Deletion of final	Deletion	Syllable reduction
consonant	2. Velar Fronting:	Cluster reduction
Cluster Reductions:	Initial	Prevocalic obstruent
Initial Stop + Liquid	Final	singleton omissions
Initial Fric + Liquid	3. Stopping:	Postvocalic obsturent
Initial /s/ clusters	Initial	singleton omissions
Final /s/ + Stop	Final	Stridency deletion
Final Liquid + Stop	4. Palatal Fronting:	Velar deviations
Final Nasal + Stop	Initial	
Weak Syllable Deletion	Final	*Miscellaneous*
Glottal Replacement	5. Liquid Simplification:	*Phonological Processes*
	Initial	Prevocalic voicing
Harmony Processes	Final	Postvocalic devoicing
Labial assimilation	6. Assimilation:	Glottal replacement
Alveolar assimilation	Progressive	Backing
Velar assimilation	Regressive	Stopping
Prevocalic voicing	7. Cluster Reduction:	Affrication
Final consonant devoicing	Initial	Deaffrication
Syllable Harmony	Final	Palatalization
	8. Unstressed Syllable	Depalatalization
Feature Contrast Processes	Deletion	Coalescence
Stopping		Epenthesis
Gliding of fricatives		Metathesis
Affrication		
Fronting		*Sonorant Deviations*
Denasalization		Liquid /l/
Gliding of liquids		Liquid /r ɚ/
Vocalization		Nasals
		Glides
		Vowels
		Assimilations
		Nasal
		Velar
		Labial
		Alveolar
		Articulatory Shifts
		Substitutions of
		/f v s z/ for /θ ð/
		Frontal lisp
		Dentalization of /t d n l/
		Lateralization
		Other Patterns

Ingram (1981)	Grunwell (1985)	Dean et al. (1990)
Deletion of Final Consonant	*Structural Simplifications*	*Systemic Processes*
1. Nasals	Weak Syllable Deletion:	Velar Fronting
2. Voiced stops	pretonic	Palato Alveolar Fronting
3. Voiceless stops	posttonic	Stopping of Fricatives
4. Voiced fricatives		Stopping of Affricates
5. Voiceless fricatives	*Final Consonant Deletion:*	Word Final Devoicing
	nasals	Context Sensitive Voicing
Reduction of Consonant Cluster	plosives	(i.e. WI)
6. Liquids	fricatives	Liquid Gliding
7. Nasals	affricates	Fricative Simplification
8. /s/ clusters	clusters - 1	($\theta \rightarrow$ f; $\eth \rightarrow$ v)
	- 2+	Backing of Alveolar Stops
Syllable deletion & Reduplication	Vocalization:	(Unusual/atypical process)
9. Reduction of disyllables	/l/	
10. Unstressed syllable deletion	other C	*Structural Processes*
11. Reduplication	Reduplication:	Final Consonant Deletion
	complete	Initial Cluster Reduction/ Deletion
Fronting	partial	Initial Consonant Deletion
12. of palatals	Consonant Harmony:	(Unusual/atypical process)
13. of velars	velar	Final Cluster Reduction/ Deletion
	alveolar	(Unusual/atypical process)
Stopping	labial	
14. of initial voiceless fricatives	manner	
15. of initial voiced fricatives	other	
16. of initial affricates	S.I. Cluster Reduction:	
	plosive + approx.	
Simplification of Liquids and Nasals	fricative + approx.	
17. Liquid Gliding	/s/ + plosive	
18. Vocalization	/s/ + nasal	
19. Denasalization	/s/ + approx.	
	/s/ + plosive + approx.	
Other Substitution Processes	*Systemic Simplifications*	
20. Deaffrication	Fronting:	
21. Deletion of initial consonants	velars	
22. Apicalization	palato-alveolars	
23. Labialization	Stopping:	
	/f/ /v/	
Assimilation Processes	/θ/ /ð/	
24. Velar assimilation	/s/ /z/	
25. Labial assimilation	/ʃ/	
26. Prevocalic voicing	/tʃ/ /dʒ/	
27. Devoicing of final cons.	/l/ /r/	

continued

Table 3–1. *Continued*

Ingram (1981)	Grunwell (1985)	Dean et al. (1990)
	Gliding:	
	/r/	
	/l/	
	fricatives	
	Context Sensitive Voicing	
	WI and WF	
	Voicing WI	
	Voicing WW	
	Devoicing WF	
	Glottal Replacement:	
	WI	
	WW	
	WF	
	Glottal Insertion	

different sets of phonological processes for the six assessment procedures. All the procedures, except Shriberg and Kwiatkowski (1980), subclassify the processes into different categories and include patterns that are not typical of normal child speech.

With regard to the classification of processes, the categories are largely defined by reference to the type of simplification the processes describe. Weiner (1979) employs the classification suggested by Ingram (1976) except that he replaces Ingram's term "substitution process" (p. 39) with the term "feature contrast processes." Ingram (1981) essentially employs the same categories: syllable structure processes, substitution processes, and assimilation. Grunwell (1985), and following her Dean, Howell, Hill, and Waters (1990) identify only two types of processes: systemic simplifications, which are substitution processes, and structural simplifications, which involve changes in syllabic structure. Reduplication and consonant harmony are included in the category of structural simplifications because phonotactically they result in simpler word structures by comparison with the adult target form of a word. Hodson (1980) employs a different classification. Her categorization is on the basis of occurrence "in the speech of children with the most severe phonological disorders" (p. 9). The basic phonological processes are those "which have been found to be prevalent" (p. 9) in the speech of such children. The miscellaneous phonological processes are not found "with the same overall pervasiveness" (p. 12) but have been observed in several children. Hodson comments that they have varying effects on intelligibility. It is in this discussion that it emerges that this is the primary factor in Hodson's categorization of processes as basic, miscellaneous and other. She comments that, "Most sonorant deviations do not seem to decrease intelligibility as much as do a number of other processes" (p. 15). Hodson's assimilations differ from Weiner's and Ingram's in that she does not include voicing processes. Her final category, articulatory shifts, involves "distortions or 'similar sounding' substitutions . . . [which] do not usually affect intelligibility greatly" (p. 19). Hodson partially supports her categorization by reference to research into the phonological systems of 60 intelligible normally developing 4-year-olds and 60 "essentially unintelligible" children between 3;0 and 8;0 (Hodson & Paden, 1981). The unintelligible children used processes that did not occur with any frequency in the pronunciation of the normally developing children. These processes were: final consonant deletion, fronting of velars, backing, syllable reduction, prevocalic voicing, and glottal replacement. They also exhibited cluster reduction, stridency deletion, stopping, and liquid deviations. It is evident therefore that Hodson's categorization is not entirely based on this single study, but also on clinical experience, as many of the processes not present in the normally developing 4-year-olds are typical of earlier stages of normal development. Most of the assessment procedures have essentially similar processes in their frameworks as can be seen on Table 3-1. These processes will be defined here using Grunwell's (1985) classification.

Structural Simplifications

Weak syllable deletion (WSD) is omission (or loss) of unstressed syllable(s) in a word of more than one syllable. Ingram (1981, p. 78) distinguishes between reduction of disyllables, (deletion of an unstressed syllable following a stressed syllable) and unstressed syllable deletion (deletion of an unstressed syllable that precedes a stressed syllable); just as Grunwell (1985, p. 54) identifies pretonic and post-tonic WSD with examples such as *banana* ['nɑnə] and *elephant* ['ɛfənt]. Hodson (1980, p. 10) and Shriberg and Kwiatkowski (1980, p. 42) do not make this distinction, although the latter only give pretonic examples. Weiner (1979, p. 3) and subsequently Grunwell (1987, p. 212) suggest the pretonic unstressed syllable is the most vulnerable. This phenomenon in child speech can clearly be construed as a natural process that reduces complexity and renders child speech patterns closer to the basic babbling patterns with regularly recurring identical syllables.

Final consonant deletion (FCD) is an apparently simple process that describes the omission of final consonants. However omissions are never as simple as they seem. For example, Hodson (1980, pp. 16–17) includes glottal replacement as an example of FCD, whereas Shriberg and Kwiatkowski (1980, p. 39) exclude glottal stops completely, as unreliable in transcription. Ingram (1981, p. 78) and Grunwell (1985, pp. 54–55) subclassify target final consonants according to manner of articulation and voicing. Hodson (1980) by default in invoking the intelligibility factor distinguishes obstruent and sonorant deletions. Weiner (1979, p. 3) does not distinguish between consonant types in his analysis, but suggests that obstruents are more vulnerable than sonorants. Examples: *bus* [bʌ], *bed* [bɛ], *bin* [bɪ].

Cluster reduction (CR) involves the deletion of one or more members of a consonant cluster—a sequence of consonants that occupy the same position in syllable structure. The primary focus is on syllable initial, especially word initial, clusters. Ingram (1976, pp. 31–34; 1981, p. 78) and Grunwell (1985, p. 58) identify different types of reduction dependent on the target constituents of the cluster. Both exemplify the same patterns; Ingram however invokes the concept of markedness in that the marked member is frequently that which is deleted. This is exemplified in the patterns of initial consonant cluster reduction:

(3) s + C → C : *smoke* [məʊk] *star* [tɑ]
plosive + approximant → plosive : *brown* [baʊn] *train* [teɪn]
clean [kin].

The opposite reduction pattern is unlikely. Both Ingram (1976) and Grunwell (1985, 1987) provide further details and discuss the patterns of cluster development, involving *feature synthesis,* such as *sl* → [ɬ] where the child's pronunciation encapsulates in one segment the features of the two targets and *epenthesis,* such as *sl* → [səl], where a vowel is inserted to break up the cluster and make it easier to pronounce. Hodson (1980) includes both these phenomena as miscellaneous processes, that is coalescence and epenthesis, respectively.

Patterns of cluster reduction in final consonant clusters are less frequently discussed. Weiner, (1979, p. 3) and Ingram (1981, p. 78) include final consonant clusters in the cluster reduction process; Hodson does by implication in sampling the following final clusters [nz; bz; ks; sk]. Grunwell (1985, pp. 54–55) includes reduction of final consonant clusters in the FCD process.

Cluster reduction is a pattern of child pronunciation that is particularly amenable to a natural phonological analysis especially when the tendency is for the so-called marked member of the target cluster to be deleted. Liquids and fricatives are evidently marked targets for children (see later); therefore Stampe's theoretical definition of a phonological process can be applied precisely in the explanation of cluster reduction: sequences of two or more consonants are more complex than single consonants; in the sequence *st*, [s] as a fricative is more complex than the plosive [t]; therefore the cluster is reduced, naturally, to [t]. It is, therefore, surprising that Stampe never discusses this phonological process.

Voicing is one of the few patterns in these clinical procedures that Stampe discusses. Ingram (1976, pp. 35–36) discusses voicing as an assimilation process, in that consonants are voiced prevocalically in anticipation of the voicing of vowels and consonants are voiceless finally in anticipation of the voicelessness of silence. Weiner (1979, p. 5), Hodson (1980, pp. 12–13), and Ingram (1981, p. 79) describe this process in a similar way. Grunwell (1985, p. 56) identifies the process as context sensitive voicing (CSV) and classifies it as a systemic simplification because of its functional consequences: the loss of the voiced/voiceless contrast such that: initial targets *p/b* → [b] and final targets *t/d* → [t]; thus [bat] could be *bat; bad; pat; pad*.

Shriberg and Kwiatkowski (1980), although acknowledging ample evidence for sound changes involving voicing differences, decided not to include voicing processes in their procedures. The reason they provide is that "our experience indicates that phonetic transcription of voicing differences is extremely unreliable" (p. 11). Phonetically this has a sound basis in fact, especially in word final position where the voicing feature is completely compromised. Nonetheless, it is important in the clinical context to decide whether or not the contrast is signalled, by whatever combination of phonetic/acoustic properties.

Reduplication, like voicing, is included in the majority of clinical procedures, except Shriberg and Kwiatkowski (1980) again, Hodson (1980) and the Metaphon Set (Dean et al., 1990). Shriberg and Kwiatkowski (1980, p. 10) exclude reduplication because it is not prevalent in their data collected from children "with moderately to severely delayed speech." Hodson's exclusion is based on a similar argument.

Definitions of this pattern are particularly unprecise. The target is a disyllabic or multisyllabic word; the child preserves or partially preserves the target syllabic structure by duplicating the prominent (i.e. usually stressed) syllable of the target word; thus *bottle* [bɒbɒ]. Weiner (1979, p. 5) calls this pattern syllable harmony. Grunwell (1985, p. 55) distinguishes between complete reduplication as in the above example and partial reduplication such as *bottle* [bɒdɒ] (vowel reduplication) and ['bɒbə] (consonant reduplication). Associated patterns include doubling and diminutives. Doubling involves the creation of a two syllable form where the target is monosyllabic, such as: *cat* ['kaka]. Diminutives involve the addition of [i] or even [Ci] as a final syllable, usually again for target monosyllables, e.g., *dog* ['dɒgi] *hi!* ['haɪdi] (Stoel-Gammon & Dunn, 1985).

In normal development, reduplication and doubling tend to co-occur with final consonant deletion (Ferguson, 1983) and may perhaps provide the basis for the development of syllable closing consonants.

Assimilation (or consonant harmony) is included in all procedures, except Metaphon. It involves patterns in children's pronunciations that manifest harmonization in the consonants in a word usually with regard to place of articulation, such as *dark* [gɑk] *table* ['beɪbʊ], or manner of articulation, such as nasality in *thumb* [niʌm] and *smell* [mɛn]. Velar harmony as in *dark* [gɑk] is commonly suggested as the most frequently occurring and therefore typical process.

In normal development, however, this pattern, like reduplication, occurs only in the very earliest stages of language development. It is therefore difficult to ascertain how typical it is. Leonard (1985, see further later) suggests that clinically it should be classified as unusual.

Vocalization was suggested by Ingram (1976, pp. 42–43) as the process whereby syllabic consonants, including nasals (e.g., *button* ['bʌtn̩]) and liquids (e.g., *bottle* ['bɒtl̩]; *cracker* ['krakɹ̩] (in an American pronunciation are realized in child speech as full vowels, without the consonants in word final position; thus *button* ['bʌtə]; *bottle* ['bɒtə]; *cracker* ['kakə]. In subsequent publications, syllabic nasals are not mentioned and only syllabic /l/ and /r/ are considered (Weiner, 1979, p. 6; Hodson, 1980, p. 16 uses the term "vowelization"; Ingram, 1981, p. 79). Shriberg and Kwiatkowski (1980, p. 41) include the possibility of vocalization in the category of liquid simplification. Grunwell, idiosyncratically, classifies vocalization as a structural simplification and not only points to the fact that vocalization results in simplified CVCV syllabic structures but also indicates that vocalization of syllabic /r/ is irrelevant in many British English accents and that vocalization of /l/ not just in syllabic contexts is typical of many accents of English. Acceptable pronunciations include, for example: *bottle* ['bɒtʊ] or ['bɒʔʊ]; *milk* [mɪʊk] or [mɪʊʔ] depending on accentual variation. Although Stampe in developing the theory of natural phonology examines issues surrounding syllabic consonants, this is never a factor on which he focuses in his theoretical exposition. In practice, the clinical relevance of vocalization is not well established because of the very important issue of accent variation.

Systemic Simplifications

Fronting is a process that is defined very specifically or more generally. As the term implies the process involves a change in the place of articulation of the target consonant to a more anterior placement. The example common to all procedures is the fronting of velar stops /k g ŋ/ to the alveolar place of articulation: [t d n]. Hodson (1980, p. 12) includes this pattern in velar deviations (a "basic process") and gives [p b m] as well as [t d n] as possible realizations. Labial realizations of target velars should probably be regarded as an unusual rather than a typical child pattern.

Several procedures include fronting of palatoalveolars /tʃ dʒ ʃ ʒ/ or palatal fronting. This follows Ingram (1976, pp. 40–41) who describes the pronunciations [t d] for these targets as involving stopping and fronting, and the pronunciations [ts dz s z] as involving just fronting.

Grunwell (1985, p. 55) takes exactly the same position as Ingram (1976). Weiner (1979, p. 5) is less specific in indicating that as well as velar stops fronting "can occur in fricatives"; the examples he gives are: /θ/ → [f] (see later); /ʃ/ → [s] (i.e., palatal fronting as defined above); /s/ → [θ] (i.e., a "lisp", or what Hodson would probably term "an articulatory shift," see later). Shriberg and Kwiatkowski (1980, p. 40) also provide a broad but different definition in indicating that palatal fronting results in any more anterior realization: alveolar, dental or bilabial; the only examples given are: /ʃ/ → [ð] and [ṣ].

Ingram (1981, p. 71) provides an alternative term for fronting of palatals, that is, depalatalization. His examples exclude the co-occurrence of stopping; that is, he only cites /tʃ dʒ ʃ ʒ/→ [ts dz s z]. Metaphon (Dean et al., 1990) restricts palatoalveolar fronting to this definition. One of Hodson's (1980) miscellaneous processes is depalatalization, with a similar definition.

It would be helpful, not least to ensure comparability across procedures, to have common definitions for these fronting processes. Restricted, specific definitions are most appropriate, such as:

A. Fronting of velar stops /kgŋ/ to alveolar placements, that is, [t d n]
B. Fronting of palatoalveolar affricates and fricatives /tʃ dʒ ʃ ʒ/ to alveolar placements, that is, [ts dz s z].

No other processes should be termed fronting.

Stopping is a process whereby target fricatives and affricates are replaced by homorganic stops. This is the definition given by Ingram,

(1976, pp. 39–40). Weiner (1979, p. 5) suggests that this is the most common of the feature contrast processes and that it frequently co-occurs with prevocalic voicing. However, he only exemplifies stopping of fricatives; in fact, in his procedure there are no processes that describe realizations of affricate targets. Once again, Shriberg and Kwiatkowski (1980, p. 40) are less specific in their definition, suggesting that stopping occurs when fricatives and affricates are replaced by any "phonemic stop" (presumably [p b t d k g]; the glottal stop is specifically excluded, as it is from their entire procedure).

Hodson's procedure analyzes these patterns differently and less concisely. The basic process stridency deletion includes the replacement of a strident by a "non-strident phoneme" (Hodson, 1980, p. 12), the example given is /s/ → [p; b; t; d; h]. In the miscellaneous processes, there is stopping that involves the substitution of stops for other consonants. It is described as a frequently occurring process that often occurs concurrently with stridency deletion. However, the examples given are: /l/ → [d]; /θ/ → [t]. It would appear from this definition that in realizations such as /s/ → [t] there are two processes effecting the same sound change. Not only is this confusing, it is theoretically unsound. Ingram (1981, pp. 78–79) restricts stopping to syllable initial position, without any explanation for this structural restriction. He also does not specify that stopping involves homorganic replacements: one of his examples does not; this is /ʃ/ → [k]. He does, however, include affricates, describing the pattern in these instances as "complete Stopping" (p. 79).

Grunwell (1985, p. 56) provides a definition of the process and specific examples of the realizations of all relevant targets. She points out that the fricatives and affricates are stopped to homorganic or *nearly* homorganic plosives:

/f/ → [p]	/v/ → [b]
/θ/ → [p/t]	/ð/ → [b/d]
/s/ → [t]	/z/ → [d]
/ʃ/ → [t]	/ʒ/ → [d]
/tʃ/ → [t]	/dʒ/ → [d]

Like Weiner, she alludes to the likely co-occurrence with the voicing process. The labial and alveolar alternative realizations of /θ ð/ are also discussed. Once again, as with the definition of fronting, this type of specific definition is more useful clinically to avoid confusion and ensure comparability.

Grunwell (1985, p. 56) also uniquely refers to stopping of the liquids /l r/ → [d]. This is based on Ingram's suggestion (1976, p. 41) that this might be an early pattern for these targets that for some children may briefly precede the more common and longer-lasting gliding (see later). One of the examples quoted from Hodson is an instance of this pattern, but she does not specifically identify it as such.

Gliding is the replacement of a liquid by a glide, such as /l/ → [j] or [w] and /r/ → [w] or [j]. Ingram (1976, pp. 41–42) identifies this as a common pattern. Weiner (1979, p. 6) follows Ingram precisely, even mentioning as does Ingram (1976) the possibility of [h] realisations of liquids being classified as instances of gliding. Weiner also refers to gliding of fricatives, identifying it as a process characteristic of atypical speech development. He states that it occurs in word initial and within word positions and that the patterns are: sibilants → [j]; other fricatives → [w].

Ingram (1981, p. 79) only mentions liquid gliding and does not refer to [h] realizations nor to gliding of fricatives. Grunwell (1985, p. 56) on the other hand includes both gliding of liquids and gliding of fricatives. For the latter, the examples given concur with the pattern suggested by Weiner. Unlike Weiner, however, Grunwell describes gliding of fricatives as an early much less common pattern.

Hodson (1980) and Shriberg and Kwiatkowski (1980) refer to gliding but from somewhat different perspectives, Hodson (pp. 15-16) includes gliding in the category sonorant deviations, alongside vowelization (see previous) and omissions. Similarly, Shriberg and Kwiatkowski (p. 41) include gliding in the process of liquid simplification that also includes vocalization (see previous). In summary, ignoring the differences in categorization, gliding of liquids is a process with an agreed on, common definition.

Other Processes

The processes discussed thus far are not only common to the clinical procedures employing the natural phonological concepts, they are also processes that are identified as typical of normal phonological development (except perhaps gliding of fricatives). In many of the procedures other processes are referred to and most often described as characteristic of disordered (or deviant) speech development. These processes are particularly relevant to the concerns of this volume. Some of these processes occur in several of the procedures. These will be discussed next.

Glottal Replacement/Realization

This is the use of the glottal stop [ʔ] as a replacement for target consonants. Ingram (1976), Weiner (1979), Hodson (1980), and Grunwell

(1985) all identify this as a pattern characteristic of disordered development; Hodson qualifying this description with "severe" (1980, p. 13). Shriberg and Kwiatkowski (1980) include this process in their list of 43 possible processes (p. 5) but exclude the glottal stop from their procedure because its transcription, they claim, is unreliable. Ingram (1981) does not mention this pattern.

Both Weiner (1979) and Hodson (1980) link the occurrence of glottal stops with deletion processes especially FCD (see previous), both requiring that a deletion as well as a glottal replacement be recorded in the analysis. Indeed, Weiner states: "We believe glottal replacement serves to mark the place of a consonant that is deleted," which implies a curious non-status for the glottal stop as a consonantal type. Grunwell (1985, pp. 56-57) simply describes the possible occurrence of glottal replacement and also mentions glottal insertion, for example *pussy* ['pʊʔsi] as a characteristic of atypical speech development.

Denasalization

Ingram (1976, p. 41) describes denasalization as an early process whereby target nasals are realized as homorganic plosives and suggests that it is not a frequent process in normal development. Weiner (1979) and Ingram (1981) include denasalization in their list of processes. Hodson (1980, p. 17) mentions non-nasal substitutions for target nasals but does not provide further details or examples. Grunwell (1985, p. 59) includes the realization of target nasals as non-nasal, usually homorganic, plosives in the list of other systemic simplifications. Examples include: *broom* [bub] *spoon* [bud].

Affrication and Deaffrication

Affrication is described by Weiner (1979, p. 5) and Hodson (1980, p. 14) as the realization of target fricatives as affricates, e.g., /s/ → [ts]. Both regard this as a transitional phase in the development of the plosive-fricative contrast. Grunwell (1985, p. 59) assesses such a pattern similarly and contrasts this with affrication of plosives, which she classifies as an unusual process, e.g., /t/ → [ts].

Deaffrication is only mentioned by Hodson (1980, p. 14) and Ingram (1981, p. 79). It involves target affricates being realized as fricatives, for example /tʃ/ → [ʃ]. Hodson suggests that it is a result of overgeneralization of a new consonant, presumably [ʃ] which can be mastered before [tʃ]. Ingram includes deaffrication in his list of four other substitution processes.

The three other substitution processes are proposed by Ingram (1981 p. 79):

■ **Deletion of initial consonants,** for example, *soup* [up]. This pattern is also included in the Metaphon set (Dean et al., 1990) where it is identified as an atypical or unusual process. This contrasts with Grunwell's inclusion of initial consonant adjunction in her set of other processes, for example *apple* ['wabʊ].

■ **Apicalization** of labial consonants, for example *pie* [taɪ] *for* [sɔ]. Although no example is provided by Ingram (1981) this process would appear to be similar to the process of tetism proposed by Grunwell (1985, p. 59) following Ingram (1976, p. 116). In tetism /f/ is is realized as [t] or [d]; it is an atypical process characteristic of disordered child speech.

■ **Labialization** of lingual consonants to labial place or articulation, for example *thumb* [fʌm]. This example, provided by Ingram (1981, p. 79), is a very common entirely normal immaturity, which may indeed be an acceptable mature pronunciation in certain accent communities. It is unfortunate that this is linked with other clearly atypical processes. Hodson (1980, p. 19) includes this pattern in articulatory shifts. By contrast Grunwell's other process of labial realizations of fricatives with examples such as /s/ → [f] or [w]; /ʃ/→ [f] are clearly atypical.

In addition, Hodson (1980) includes: **Backing** of non-back targets as an infrequent process that "devastates intelligibility" according to Hodson (p. 13). As mentioned, Hodson's definitions tend to be nonspecific; her example *tub* [kʌg] suggests both target alveolars and labials may be involved.

Grunwell (1985, p. 59; and following her, Dean et al., 1990), on the other hand, is quite specific that backing involves the realization of target alveolars as velars, that is, *tap* [kap]—the opposite of velar fronting. Grunwell (1985, p. 59) also includes backing in terminations, where velar consonants are used for a variety of targets in word final position, such as *mouse* [maʊk] *glove* [dʌg].

Hodson's (1980) other processes are:

■ Palatalization of stridents: /s/ → [sʲ] or [ʃ] and clusters /gr/ → [dʒ]

■ Glide omissions and substitutions, vowel deviations and various articulatory shifts for which no specific examples are provided.

Grunwell (1985) lists a number of other processes:

- Vocalic support for final consonants and vowel insertion before a final consonant, both of which may be iatrogenic: *bed* ['bɛdə] *race* ['weɪəs].
- Dissimilation, perseveration and metathesis that involve sound sequences, with examples respectively: *pipe* [baɪt], *lipstick* ['lɪptɪp], *elephant* ['ɛfələnt]. (Hodson also mentions metathesis [1980, p. 15]).
- Lateral realizations of sibilants, such as /s/ → [ɬ]
- Weakening (or spirantization) of plosives, such as /p/ → [f] /t/ → [s].

These are all to be regarded as less common processes; some are possibly atypical of normal development.

Unusual Phonological Processes

Leonard (1985) specifically defined unusual phonological processes that had been previously identified in the speech of children with phonological disorders who did not have identifiable physical, physiological, or auditory deficiencies. Three categories of phonological behavior are identified, the third of which will not be considered in this discussion. (That category deals with phonetic phenomena that are imperceptible to adult listeners, but through acoustic analysis are revealed as evidence that in a child's speech a contrast is regularly signalled by phonetic properties that can be directly related to subphonemic phenomena in the target pronunciations, such as Voice Onset Time for initial stops and vowel length for final stops.)

Leonard's two other categories of unusual phonological behaviors are:

1. Salient but unusual sound changes with readily detectable systematicity.
2. Salient but unusual sound changes with less readily detectable systematicity.

In support of this classification Leonard cites examples from phonologically oriented studies of disordered child speech published primarily in the period from 1975 to 1985. Table 3–2 exemplifies the categories using data from one exceptionally disordered child subject (see also Grunwell, 1992a).

Table 3–2. Unusual phonological behavior: M.T. 3;11.

1. Salient but Unusual Sound Changes with Readily Detectable Systematicity
   —*Early Sounds replaced by late sounds*
   /p/: [k] pencil ['kɛnzəɫ] teapot ['sikɒʔ]
   —*Additions to adult forms*
   (a) Vocalizations
   clouds ['ɬaʊwi] tights ['taɪʔi] watch ['jɒʔi]
   (b) initial consonant adjunction
   on [lɒ] up [lʌ] umbrella [lu'lɛlə]
   ice cream ['saɪˌn̥ᶠki]
   —*Use of sounds absent from model language*
   (a) [ɬ] clock [ɬɒp] clouds ['ɬaʊwi]
   plate [ɬleɪk] playground ['ɬleɪdaʊ]
   (b) [ʃ] mouse [ʃaʊ] mouth [ʃaʊ]
   —*Use of sounds absent from natural languages*

[n̥ᶠ]	soft	[n̥ᶠdɒ]	soldier	['n̥ᶠtoʊjə]
	sand	[n̥ᶠkan;n̥ᶠsdan]		
	shoe	[n̥ᶠgu]	sugar	['n̥ᶠgʊgə]
	shop	[n̥ᶠskɒ]	shaving	['n̥ᶠdeɪji]
	spade	[n̥ᶠteɪ]	splash	['n̥ᶠtla]
	spoon	[n̥ᶠsku]	spring	[n̥ᶠnɪn]
	star	[n̥ᶠstɑ]	string	['n̥ᶠtɪn]
	scarf	[n̥ᶠgɑ]	scribble	['n̥ᶠbɪbɫ]
	square	[n̥ᶠgɛə]		
	smoke	[n̥ᶠmoʊk]	snake	[n̥ᶠneɪ]

   [n̥ᶠ]—Voiceless alveolar nasal with audible nasal friction.

2. Salient but Unusual Sound Changes with Less Readily Detectable Systematicity
   —*Assimilations*
   (a) *Reduplications*

birthday	['dɜdeɪ]	chimney	['kɪki]
cupboard	['kʌkə]	ladder	['lala]
drinking	['gɪgi]	rainbow	['weɪwoʊ]
wardrobe	['wɔwoʊ]	window	['nɪnoʊ]

   (b) *Consonant harmony*

flag	[kag]	gate	[geɪg]
ring	[nɪn]		

   —*Metathesis*

bag	[ga]	bucket	['gʊʔɪ]
hedgehog	['jɛgɒ]	motorbike	['noʊgaɪ]
orange	['ɒni:]	garden	['ganə]

   —*Syllable structure deletions*
   (a) *Post-tonic weak syllable deletion*

baby	[beɪ]	bottle	[gɒɫ]
dinosaur	['daɪn̥ᶠθɔ]	caravan	['kaŋˌna]
vinegar	['bɪdə]	finger	[n̥ᶠgə]

   (b) *Within-word consonant deletion*

apple	['au]	laughing	['lɑːi]
sleeping	[ɬliːɪ]	caterpillar	['kaɪsioʊ]

**Salient but Unusual Sound Changes
With Readily Detectable Systematicity**

These are atypical substitution patterns, such as:

- Early sounds replaced by late sounds;
- Additions to adult forms, such as additional consonant adjunction: see Table 3–2;
- Use of sounds absent from the model language; and
- Use of sounds absent from natural language.

**Salient But Unusual Sound Changes With
Less Readily Detectable Systematicity**

These are essentially assimilative or structural changes, some of which have been identified in previous assessments as typical of normal phonological development. Leonard (1985) cites examples of older children who continue to exhibit such patterns in their pronunciation systems. These are:

- Assimilations, both reduplications and consonant harmony;
- Metathesis; and
- Syllable structure deletions, such as posttonic weak syllable deletion and within-word consonant deletion. (see Table 3–2).

Innate Universal Processes?

It will be evident to the reader that the clinical procedures, phonological processes, and examples described thus far refer only to English. This is because the major sources of published studies on phonological development and disorders are in English about English-speaking children. However, there are some published reports, using the phonological process framework, that describe the characteristics of speech development and speech disorders in children learning languages other than English. With some important qualifications, these reports lend credence to the theory of natural phonology, in that the phonological processes are in some sense innate and therefore universal, because of the phonetic basis of speech.

Ingram (1979, 1986) cites examples from French, Hungarian, Polish, Estonian, German, and Romanian. These examples illustrate the occurrence of stopping, fronting, gliding, voicing, consonant harmony, cluster reduction, final consonant deletion, syllable deletion and reduplication in languages other than English. They provide evidence that these are characteristics of speech development that are common to all children, and are not language specific.

Nettelbladt (1983) appears to be one of the first published studies that applied the phonological process framework to another language: Swedish. She reports on 10 Swedish-speaking children with "dysphonology" and one normally developing subject. Her analyses are comprehensive, including vowels and suprasegmental characteristics. The phonological process analysis used is not aligned specifically with any pre-existing English-based framework; however, common processes such as syllable deletion, reduplication, consonant harmony, and cluster reduction are identified. There are also processes with definitions that do not easily match other frameworks; for example H-zation, which describes the use of [h] for other consonants, e.g. /t; s; r; ʃ/. Nettelbladt (1983) presents extremely interesting findings about the identification of different types of dysphonology/developmental phonological disorders. In relation to this chapter, her study illustrates the applicability of process analysis, as well as the need to be language sensitive.

This conclusion is replicated in a study of Italian children (Bortolini & Leonard, 1991; see also Leonard, Devescovi, & Ossella, 1987). Bortolini and Leonard describe occurrences of common patterns, such as cluster reduction, in both normal and phonologically disordered children and stopping and fronting in phonologically disordered children. There were, however, frequently occurring patterns that clearly reflected a sensitivity to the ambient language, particularly in regard to liquid realisations. Italian /r/ is a trill; gliding was completely absent; the most common child realization was [l]. Weak syllable deletion was another frequent process, reflecting the high proportion of polysyllabic words in Italian. Although this study emphasizes the language-sensitive nature of phonological acquisition, it also illustrates the presence of universal tendencies.

The studies of Yavas and Lamprecht (1988) and So and Dodd (1994) confirm this point. Yavas and Lamprecht report a study of four phonologically disordered Portuguese-speaking children. Their subjects evidence several of the already identified processes, such as cluster reduction and liquid subsitutions. They also conform to the characterisitics of developmental phonological disability, showing persisting normal processes, chronological mismatch and so on (see further later). However, there appear to be some language-specific aspects of the pronunciation patterns; these are the occurrence of context-free obstruent devoicing, the almost complete nonexistence of fricative stopping, and the lack of glottal replacements.

So and Dodd (1994) report the patterns of 17 phonologically disordered Cantonese-speaking children. Their study revealed the presence of many well-attested patterns such as stopping, fronting, final consonant deletion, and cluster reduction. They also identify some unusual patterns including the low frequency of gliding, word initial consonant deletion, backing of alveolar plosives, backing word final, and the use of [h] for aspirated plosives and /s/. While these unusual processes may be to some extent language-sensitive, they have also been previously identified as probably atypical patterns. Grunwell (1985) identifies initial consonant deletion and backing as unusual. Nettelbladt (1983) also describes an [h] substitution pattern.

There is clearly a need for studies of children who speak a much greater variety of languages. Nonetheless, from the information available, it is clear that phonological process analysis is a viable cross-linguistic procedure for the description and assessment of child speech and child speech disorders. Using this framework, common normal patterns are identified, as well as language-specific, typically disordered, and idiosyncratic patterns.

Vowels

Vowels and vowel development feature hardly at all in the prime sources for the procedures of natural phonology. Ingram (1976/89) provides a description of the early stages of vowel development and mentions some processes involving vowels such as consonant–vowel harmony (see also Grunwell, 1981b, 1987) and vowel assimilation. More recently there have been a small number of published studies of disordered vowel systems (Gibbon, Shockey & Reid 1992; Penney, Fee & Dowdle 1994; Pollock & Keiser 1990; Pollock & Hall 1991; Reynolds 1990; Stoel-Gammon & Herrington 1990). These case studies, most especially Reynolds, show the influence of process analysis. He seeks to identify patterns in vowel disorders and parallels with consonantal patterns. The key patterns Reynolds (1990) describes are:

- ■ **Lowering** of mid front vowels: /ɛ/ to [a] (also noted by Stoel-Gammon & Herrington, 1990).
- ■ **Fronting** of low back vowels to [a], (also noted by Penney, Fee, & Dowdle, 1994; Pollock & Hall, 1990 report the opposite).
- ■ **Diphthong Reduction** to monophthong: /eɪ/) → [a]) (Pollock & Hall, 1991, and Gibbon et al., 1992, also report this pattern).

Reynolds (1990) observes that these patterns conspire to maximize the occurrence of open vowels (compare with systematic sound preference; see later discussion). As such they also involve loss of contrasts and are therefore similar to consonantal processes.

There are in fact as many differences as similarities between these few studies of vowel disorders. Once again it is clear that an approach that seeks to identify simplification patterns is potentially fruitful, but that many more studies are required to construct a definitive and diagnostic description of disordered vowel systems.

Ordering of Processes

The range of natural phonological processes identified and/or assessed by clinical investigations have been described in the preceding sections. One issue that has not been discussed which formed the focus of the original presentations of the theoretical approach is the ordering, or alternatively, the co-occurrence of these processes. It would appear that, with the exception of Shriberg and Kwiatkowski (1980), the processes are regarded as co-occurring, such that, for example:

- *sky*: [taɪ] involves co-occurring cluster reduction and velar fronting

as does also

- *cry*: [taɪ].

Shriberg and Kwiatkowski, on the other hand, restrict the conventions of their analysis such that any sound change is attributed to only one process (1980, p. 12). This runs counter to Stampe's original theoretical position, in which every sound change has identifiable phonetic causalities. Describing the two quoted examples as involving only one phonological process each, conceals the *two common* phonetic causalities of both patterns.

CLINICAL EVALUATION

It is evident from the preceding outline of the descriptive assessment procedures that applying the concept of natural phonological process to clinical data provides a basis for identifying the patterns in the data, that is, the systematic relationships between the target pronunciations and those of the client (usually a child) being assessed. The identification of patterns in itself is an important clinical finding as it indicates that there are regularities in what has been deemed "disordered phonology."

Phonological process analysis is not unique in highlighting this consequence of applying phonological concepts in the analysis of clinical data (see preceding chapters). However, the assessment procedures developed from the basis of natural phonology not only identify patterns, they also classify patterns. These classifications enable clinicians to identify similarities and differences between patterns and to examine the phonological consequences of different patterns, which co-occur or interact. Thus it is important to differentiate between processes with structural and systemic implications, such as cluster reduction and fronting, and then to discover the phonological consequences when they co-occur, as in the quoted example of *sky* [taɪ] and *cry* [taɪ]. Similarly, it is important to identify the phonological consequences when two different systemic processes co-occur, such as fronting of velars and stopping of fricatives and affricates, so that:

$$/\text{k}/ \rightarrow [\text{t}]$$

and

$$\left.\begin{array}{l}/\text{s}/ \\ /\int/ \\ /\text{t}\int/\end{array}\right\} \rightarrow [\text{t}]$$

Phonological process analysis also potentially provides the basis to differentiate between typical normal patterns in speech development and atypical patterns. There is, however, a problem in defining atypical, or unusual, or idiosyncratic, patterns as they have been called. As has been indicated in the preceding section there is not total agreement as to what are the typical patterns and which patterns are atypical. Ingram (1981), for example, makes no such distinction—although this is consistent with his view "that children with phonological delay do not exhibit unique or different processes as much as the persistence or use of processes that normal children rarely use, or lose at an early age" (p. 103). Weiner (1979), on the other hand, distinguishes between patterns that are developmentally normal and patterns typical of developmental phonological disorders in his description of the processes, but not in his classification of the processes. Hodson (1980) adopts a similar approach. Shriberg and Kwiatkowski (1980) in fact only include developmentally normal processes, even though the body of data they used was taken from children with "delayed speech" (p. 9).

The problem with defining a process as atypical or idiosyncratic is that one cannot assert or prove that it has or will never occur in the speech of a child who ultimately develops speech normally. For example, Grunwell (1981b, pp. 121–123, 1987, pp. 239–241) illustrates a "deviant process" of glottal stop insertion and apical substitution:

(4) *candle* ['taʔsʊ]   *finger* ['fɪʔsʊ];

but in so doing refers to a paper reporting a similar process in normal development (Priestly, 1977), where the process was limited and short-lived. The definition of what might be considered an unusual process therefore needs to be carefully constructed (see further later).

To allow for the possible occurrence of other unusual processes it is important that a clinical assessment procedure be open-ended. Weiner (1979) intends his procedure to be so and suggests that with experience clinicians will be able better to recognize unusual processes. Unfortunately he does not provide specific examples and the format of the procedure does not lend itself to an open-ended approach. Hodson (1980) allows for the possibility of "other patterns preferences" (pp. 20–21) including as examples reduplications, nasalization, and denasalization, among others. Shriberg and Kwiatkowski's (1980) set of processes is, by definition, not open-ended (see previous discussion). Grunwell's (1985) is definitely open-ended with an illustrative list of other processes that was described in the previous section. Ingram's (1981) procedure could be open-ended, but he does not specifically discuss this issue. Metaphon (Dean et al., 1990) has a deliberately restricted set of processes, but users are encouraged to identify the occurrence of other processes not included in the set.

Given the origins of phonological process analysis in the analysis of normal speech development, the approach clearly has diagnostic potential in the clinical context. To an extent this has already been discussed in the descriptions of the different processes and the identification of those patterns that have been observed in children with delayed or disordered speech development. There is also, however, the dimension of developmental progress that needs to be assessed. Shriberg and Kwiatkowski (1980) describe stages in normal development, but Grunwell (1985) provides a more formal framework for a developmental assessment. This is based on Grunwell (1981a; see also 1987, pp. 228–231) in which a chronology of phonological processes (see Table 3–3) is presented. The sources employed in the compilation of this chronology were not confined to phonologically oriented studies of speech development; the results of studies of speech development with a variety of theoretical and applied backgrounds have been translated into the framework of phonological processes (see Grunwell, 1981a).

Table 3–3. Chronology of phonological processes.

Process	2;0–2;6	2;6–3;0	3;0–3;6	3;6–4;0	4;0–4;6	4;6–5;0	5;0→
Weak Syllable Deletion	▰▰▰	▰▰▰	▰ ▰ ▰ ▰				
Final Consonant Deletion	▰▰▰	▰ ▰ ▰ ▰					
Reduplication	▰ ▰ ▰						
Consonant Harmony	▰▰	▰ ▰ ▰					
Cluster Reduction (Initial)							
obstruent + approximant	▰▰▰	▰ ▰ ▰ ▰ ▰	▰ ▰ ▰				
/s/ + consonant	▰▰▰	▰▰▰	▰ ▰ ▰				
Stopping							
/f/	▰ ▰ ▰ ▰	▰ ▰ ▰					
/v/		▰ ▰ ▰ ▰	▰ ▰ ▰ ▰				
/θ/		/θ/→ [f] ▰ ▰	▰▰▰▰	▰▰▰	▰ ▰ ▰ ▰	▰ ▰ ▰	▰ ▰ ▰
/ð/				/ð/→[d] or [v] ▰▰▰	▰▰▰	▰ ▰ ▰	▰ ▰ ▰
/s/	▰▰	▰ ▰ ▰ ▰ ▰					
/z/		▰ ▰ ▰ ▰ ▰					
/ʃ/	Fronting "[s] type" ▰▰			▰ ▰ ▰	▰ ▰ ▰		
/tʃ, dʒ/		Fronting [ts; dz] ▰ ▰ ▰ ▰ ▰	▰ ▰ ▰ ▰				
Fronting /k, g, ŋ/		▰ ▰ ▰ ▰ ▰					
Gliding /r/ → [w]	▰▰▰	▰ ▰ ▰ ▰ ▰	▰▰▰	▰▰▰	▰▰▰	▰▰▰	▰ ▰ ▰
Context-sensitive Voicing	▰▰	▰ ▰ ▰ ▰					

This framework for a developmental diagnosis has led to the identification of three potential developmental differences (Grunwell, 1985, p. 92):

- ■ Delayed
- ■ Uneven
- ■ Deviant

With reference to the diagnostic indicators provided by a phonological process analysis, five characteristics of disordered phonological development can be identified (Grunwell, 1981b, 1985, 1987, 1988; Stoel-Gammon & Dunn, 1985):

- Persisting normal processes
- Chronological mismatch
- Unusual processes
- Variable use of processes
- Systematic sound preference

Persisting normal processes are normal phonological processes that remain in a child's pronunciation patterns long after the age at which they would be expected to have been "suppressed," such as fronting of velars present in the speech of a child of 3;6–3;9. If the processes evidenced in a data sample are all normal and are homogeneous in terms of their chronology, then it is clear that a child's phonological development is delayed to a greater or lesser extent, depending on his or her age, or is "arrested" at a particular stage of development.

Chronological mismatch is the co-occurrence of some of the earliest normal simplifying processes with some patterns of pronunciation characteristic of later stages in phonological development, such as fronting of velars and the development of word initial clusters present in the speech of a child aged 3;6–3;9. Such uneven progress is suggestive of disrupted or literally "dis-ordered" development.

Unusual processes are apparently simplifying patterns that have been rarely attested in normal speech development or that appear to be different from normal developmental processes and may, therefore, be idiosyncratic. As indicated above, this definition is carefully constructed so as not to exclude the possibility that a child who subsequently exhibits normal developmental achievements might display apparently unusual patterns for a short period of time.

Variable use of processes occurs when more than one simplifying process routinely operates with the same target type of structure, so that the child's realizations are variable and unpredictable: *pie* [baɪ] *pour* [pɔ]. This variability is potentially progressive in that it entails the possible development of target contrast. Variability is abnormal when it is not potentially progressive:

rake [leɪk]	*rabbit* [abɪt]
ring [wɪŋ]	*red* [oɛd]

Systematic sound preference occurs when one type of consonant is used for a large range of different target types. Often several different processes can be identified as resulting in a massive reduction of the phonological contrasts in a child's system: the processes "conspire" to "collapse" the adult system of contrasts to the one phone the child prefers to use in his or her pronunciation patterns (i.e., what might be called a "favorite articulation"):

- Fronting and voicing of /k/;
- Fronting of /g/;
- Stopping and voicing of /θ s ʃ tʃ/;
- Stopping of /ð z ʒ dʒ/;
- Voicing of /t/;

Cluster reduction involving these targets; the co-occurrence of all these processes thus results in systematic sound preference for [d].

The resultant massive lack of contrasts is clearly indicative of a severe phonological learning disability in a child who has developed in other aspects of language such as the lexicon and grammar beyond the earliest stages of language development. These processes only co-occur normally up to about 2;6.

These characteristics are most frequently applied in clinical diagnosis when there are no co-occurring anatomical or physiological conditions. However, as Ingram (1976) and Grunwell (1990) demonstrate, phonological process analysis is amenable to other applications. The naturalness of other phonologies can be identified (see quotation from Harris & Cottam, 1985). In addition, as children are developing pronunciation patterns in the context of an identifiable disability, there is likely to be an interaction between the normal pattern of development and the effects of the anatomical and/or physiological condition. For example, there is an identified tendency of backing in "cleft palate speech," which is the opposite of "normal fronting of velars"; alongside this tendency it is likely that children with repaired cleft palate will continue to evidence patterns of normal immaturities such as stopping of fricatives and affricates and gliding of liquids (Russell & Grunwell, 1993)[1].

TREATMENT IMPLICATIONS

The purpose of carrying out a phonologically based assessment procedure is to provide information for planning treatment: the aims of a treatment program are determined by the findings of the assessment.

---

[1]This chapter concentrates exclusively on the application of natural phonology to the analysis of disordered child speech. There are only three publications in which this approach has been used in the analysis of acquired speech disorders (Crary & Fokes, 1980; Edwards & Shriberg, 1983; Klich, Ireland, & Weidner, 1979). The primary focus in all three reports is to demonstrate that this analytical approach is capable of handling this kind of data, which it clearly is.

Hodson and Paden (1983, 1991) and Dean, Howell, Hill, and Waters, (1990) most clearly identify the relationship between the assessment procedure and a treatment program. Treatment focuses on the patterns of errors identified by the process analysis. Furthermore, it is assumed that generalization or carry-over from one instance of a pattern to another will occur. Treatment planning in the context of phonological process analysis can also be associated with a developmental framework, in that treatment programs can be planned by reference to developmental stages (e.g., see Grunwell, 1992b). There would appear to be no close relationship between the theoretical basis of natural phonology and its applications in treatment planning apart from the identification of patterns in child speech.

Conclusions

Natural phonology has been extremely successful in providing the basis for analytical and descriptive assessment procedures in the clinical evaluation of children's speech disorders. These procedures, while based on the theoretical approach propounded by David Stampe, are rarely related to his theory of phonology. Ingram (1976, p. 49) explicitly rejects Stampe's view that children "know" all the details of the form of the adult pronunciation. Ingram proposes that children's pronunciation patterns are determined by perceptual, organizational, and production constraints. This is a view shared by Leonard (1985) and Grunwell (1990). Schwartz (1984) also refutes Stampe's position, while Weiner (1984) in the same volume appears to uphold Stampe's position.

These are clearly important issues but they are beyond the scope of clinical phonological analyses. They can be addressed only in the context of a psycholinguistic investigation of pronunciation development (Spencer, 1985). Despite the discussions mentioned in the preceding paragraph, no such investigation has been undertaken.

Natural phonology, notwithstanding the discontinuity between theory and practice highlighted in this chapter, has provided the descriptive framework for appropriate clinical assessments that identify the common characteristics of developmental phonological disorders and those characteristics that are developmentally typical. These assessments are also potentially open-ended and therefore facilitate the description of developmentally atypical patterns. Most important of all, this approach to phonological assessment has consistently focused upon the necessity to identify phonologically determined patterns in clinical speech data.

REFERENCES

Bortolini, U., & Leonard, L. B. (1991). The speech of phonologically disordered children acquiring Italian. *Clinical Linguistics and Phonetics, 5,* 1–12

Crary, M. A., & Fokes, J. (1980). Phonological processes in apraxia of speech: A systemic simplification of articulatory performance. *Aphasia, Apraxia, Agnosia, 4,* 1–13.

Dean, E., Howell, J., Hill, A., & Waters, D. (1990). *Metaphon resource pack.* Windsor: NFER-Nelson.

Dinnsen, D. A. (Ed.). (1979). *Current approaches to phonological theory.* Bloomington: Indiana University Press.

Donegan, P. J., & Stampe, D. (1979). The study of natural phonology. In D. A. Dinnsen (Ed.), *Current approaches to phonological theory* (pp. 126–173). Bloomington: Indiana University Press.

Edwards, M. L., & Bernhardt, B. (1973). *Phonological analysis of the speech of four children with language disorders.* Unpublished paper, see Ingram, D. (1976).

Edwards, M. L., & Shriberg, L. D. (1983). *Phonology: Applications in communicative disorders.* San Diego: College-Hill Press.

Ferguson, C. A. (1983). Reduplication in child phonology. *Journal of Child Language , 10,* 239–243.

Gibbon, F., Shockey, L., & Reid, J. (1992). Description and treatment of abnormal vowels. *Child Language Teaching and Therapy, 8,* 30–59.

Grammont, M. (1933). *Traité de phonetique.* Paris: Librairie Delagrave.

Grunwell, P. (1981a). The development of phonology: A descriptive profile. *First Language, 3,* 161–191.

Grunwell, P. (1981b). *The nature of phonological disability in children.* London: Academic Press.

Grunwell, P. (1985). *Phonological assessment of child speech.* Windsor: NFER-Nelson.

Grunwell, P. (1987). *Clinical phonology,* 2nd ed. London: Chapman & Hall.

Grunwell, P. (1988). Phonological assessment, evaluation and explanation of speech disorders in children. [A tutorial review]. *Clinical Linguistics and Phonetics, 2,* 221–252.

Grunwell, P. (Ed.). (1990). *Developmental speech disorders.* Edinburgh: Churchill Livingstone; now London: Whurr.

Grunwell, P. (1992a). Assessment of child phonology in the clinical context. In C. A. Ferguson, L. Menn, & C. Stoel-Gammon (Eds.), *Phonological development: Models, research, implications* (pp. 457–483). Timonium, MD: York Press.

Grunwell, P. (1992b). Principled decision-making in the remediation of children with developmental phonological disorders. In P. Fletcher & D. Hall (Eds.), *Specific speech and language disorders in children* (pp. 215–240). London: Whurr.

Harris, J., & Cottam, P. (1985). Phonetic features and phonological features in speech assessment. *British Journal of Disorders of Communication, 20,* 61–74.

Hodson, B. W. (1980). *The assessment of phonological processes.* Danville, IL: Interstate Inc.

Hodson, B. W. (1982). Remediation of speech patterns associated with low levels of phonological performance. In M. A. Crary (Ed.), *Phonological intervention, concepts and procedures* (pp. 97–115). San Diego: College-Hill Press.

Hodson, B. W., & Paden, E. P. (1981). Phonological processes which characterize unintelligible and intelligible speech in early childhood. *Journal of Speech and Hearing Disorders, 46,* 369–373.

Hodson, B. W., & Paden, E. P. (1983). *Targetting intelligible speech.* San Diego: College-Hill Press.

Hodson, B. W., & Paden, E. P. (1991). *Targetting intelligible speech,* 2nd ed. Austin, TX: Pro-Ed.

Householder, F. W. (1979). How different are they? In D. A. Dinnsen (Ed.), *Current approaches to phonological theory* (pp. 252–264). Bloomington: Indiana University Press.

Howell, J., & Dean, E. (1991). *Treating phonological disorders in children: Metaphon—Theory to practice.* Kibworth: Far Communications; now London: Whurr.

Ingram, D. (1976). *Phonological disability in children.* London: Edward Arnold. (2nd ed. 1989). London: Cole & Whurr.)

Ingram, D. (1979). Phonological development: Production. In P. Fletcher & M. Garman (Eds.), *Language acquisition* (pp. 133–148). Cambridge: Cambridge University Press.

Ingram, D. (1981). *Procedures for the phonological analysis of children's language.* Baltimore: University Park Press.

Ingram, D. (1986). Phonological development: Production. In P. Fletcher & M. Garman (Eds.). *Language acquisition,* 2nd ed. (pp. 223–239). Cambridge: Cambridge University Press.

Jakobson, R. (1941). *Kinderspräche, Aphasie und allgemeine Lautgesetze.* In translation (1968) *Child language, aphasia and phonological universals.* The Hague: Mouton.

Jespersen, O. (1964). *Language: Its nature, development and origin.* New York: W. W. Norton.

Kiparsky, P. , & Menn, L. (1977). On the acquisition of phonology. In J. Macnamara (Ed.), *Language learning and thought* (pp. 47–78). New York: Academic Press.

Klich, R. J., Ireland, J. V., & Weidner, W. E. (1979). Articulatory and phonological aspects of consonant substitutions in apraxia of speech. *Cortex, 15,* 451–470.

Leonard, L. B. (1985). Unusual and subtle phonological behavior in the speech of phonologically disordered children. *Journal of Speech and Hearing Disorders, 50,* 4–13.

Leonard, L. B., Devescovi, A., & Ossella, T. (1987). Context-sensitive phonological patterns in children with poor intelligibility. *Child Language Teaching and Therapy, 3,* 125–132.

Locke, J. L. (1983a). Clinical phonology: the explanation and treatment of speech sound disorders. *Journal of Speech and Hearing Disorders, 48,* 339–341.

Locke, J. L. (1983b). *Phonological acquisition and change.* New York: Academic Press.

McCawley, J. D. (1979) Comments. In D. A. Dinnsen (Ed.). *Current approaches to phonological theory* (pp. 294–302). Bloomington: Indiana University Press.

Nettelbladt, U. (1983). *Developmental studies of dysphonology in children.* Lund: CWK Gleerup.

Oller, D. K. (1973). Regularities in abnormal child phonology. *Journal of Speech and Hearing Disorders, 38,* 35–46.

Passy, P. (1890). *Etude sur les changements phonètiques et leurs caractères.* Paris: Librairie Firmin-Didot.

Penney, G., Fee, E. J., & Dowdle, C. (1994). Vowel assessment and remediation: A case study. *Child Language Teaching and Therapy, 10,* 47–66.

Pollock, K. E., & Hall, P. K. (1991). An analysis of the vowel misarticulations of five children with developmental apraxia of speech. *Clinical Linguistics and Phonetics, 5,* 207–224.

Pollock, K. E. , & Keiser, N. J. (1990). An examination of vowel errors in phonologically disordered children. *Clinical Linguistics and Phonetics, 4,* 161–178.

Priestly, T. M. S. (1977). One idiosyncratic strategy in the acquisition of phonology. *Journal of Child Language, 4,* 45–65.

Reynolds, J. (1990). Abnormal vowel patterns: Some data and a hypothesis. *British Journal of Disorders of Communication, 25,* 115–148.

Russell, J., & Grunwell, P. (1993). Speech development in children with cleft lip and palate. In P. Grunwell (Ed.), *Analysing cleft palate speech* (pp. 19–47). London: Whurr.

Sapir, E. (1921). *Language.* New York: Harcourt Brace.

Sapir, E. (1933). The psychological reality of phonemes. *Journal de Psychologie Normale et Pathologique, 30,* 247–265. [Reprinted in: M. Joos (Ed.) *Readings in Linguistics I.,* 4th ed. Chicago: University of Chicago Press].

Schwartz, R. G. (1984). The phonologic system: Normal acquisition. In J. M. Costello (Ed.), *Speech disorders in children* (pp. 25–74). Windsor: NFER-Nelson.

Shriberg, L. D. (1982). Diagnostic assessment of developmental phonological disorders. In M. A. Crary (Ed.), *Phonological intervention, concepts and procedures* (pp. 35–60). San Diego: College-Hill Press.

Shriberg, L. D., & Kwiatkowski, J. (1980). *Natural process analysis.* New York: John Wiley.

Smith, N. V. (1973). *The acquisition of phonology: A case study.* Cambridge: Cambridge University Press.

So, L. K. H., & Dodd, B. J. (1994). Phonologically disordered Cantonese-speaking children. *Clinical Linguistics and Phonetics, 8,* 235–255.

Spencer, A. (1985). A phonological theory of phonological development. In M. J. Ball (Ed.), *Theoretical linguistics and disordered language* (pp. 115–151). London: Croom Helm.

Stampe, D. (1969). The acquisition of phonetic representation. *Papers from the Fifth Regional Meeting of the Chicago Linguistic Circle.* Chicago: University of Chicago Department of Linguistics.

Stampe, D. (1979). *A dissertation on natural phonology.* New York: Garland Publishing Inc.

Stoel-Gammon, C., & Dunn, C. (1985). *Normal and disordered phonology in chil-*

dren. Baltimore: University Park Press.

Stoel-Gammon, C. , & Herrington, P. B. (1990). Vowel systems of normally developing and phonologically disordered children. *Clinical Linguistics and Phonetics, 4*, 145-160.

Sweet, H. (1877). *Handbook of phonetics*. Oxford: Clarendon Press.

Weiner, F. F. (1979). *Phonological process analysis*. Baltimore: University Park Press.

Weiner, F. F. (1984). A phonologic approach to assessment and treatment. In J. M. Costello (Ed.), *Speech disorders in children* (pp. 75–91). Windsor: NFER-Nelson.

Yavas, M., & Lamprecht, R. (1988). Processes and intelligibility in disordered phonology. *Clinical Linguistics and Phonetics, 2*, 329–345.

CHAPTER

4

Nonsegmental Phonologies

DANIEL A. DINNSEN

Current conceptions of phonological structure and representations have changed considerably from those adopted by earlier segment-based frameworks, including, among others, those of early generative theory (e.g., Chomsky & Halle, 1968). An essential claim of these earlier frameworks has been that phonological representations are linear—that is, constituted by a string of discrete segments (systematic phonemes), each analyzable as an unstructured bundle of distinctive features. A further claim has been that a common set of features is attributed to all segments and that each feature is specified for a "+" or "−" coefficient value, yielding a fully specified representation. A limiting consequence of this for phonological rules is that it is only whole segments that can be deleted or added, and that the only other possible modification to a segment is achieved by changing the coefficient value of one or more features. Because all segments are equally complex under this view, there would be no reason to expect any one segment over another to be deleted, added, or modified. Also, because all features of a segment are equal and unstructured, there is no reason to expect any one group of features over another to affect or be affected by any given phonological rule.

Finally, because the notions "segment" and "feature" are inseparable, no phonological rule could operate on one without affecting the other. Continuing investigations of fully developed languages have revealed a variety of phenomena that challenge these earlier segment-based approaches in favor of what might be termed **nonsegmental phonologies**. In these more recent frameworks, segments and features are independent, features are organized into structured bundles, and representations are minimally specified. The purpose of this chapter is twofold: (a) to sketch the broad outlines of and motivation for three general nonsegmental frameworks, namely autosegmental phonology, feature geometry, and underspecification theory, and (b) to illustrate some of the implications of these frameworks for the characterization of developing sound systems with special emphasis on phonological disorders and their treatment.

THEORETICAL FRAMEWORKS: MOTIVATION AND FORMALISM

Autosegmental Phonology

A range of phenomena in fully developed languages originally motivated the introduction of autosegmental representations (e.g., Goldsmith, 1979). Autosegmental representations are fundamentally different from conventional segmental representations in that features can be represented on one tier and segments on another parallel tier, resulting in a multilayered representation. This allows for representation of a number of empirically distinct relationships between features and segments. A single feature may be associated with one or more segments or possibly even no segment. Likewise, a single segment may be associated with a single feature, a linear sequence of features, or even no feature. The display in (1) schematizes the range of possibilities. A segment is designated as "x," a feature as "F," and the association between a feature and segment by a solid line.

(1) Autosegmental relationships between segments and features

   a. One to one

   x
   |
   [+F]

b. One to many (assimilation)

[+F]

c. Many to one (contour tones)

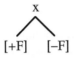

[+F]   [−F]

d. One to none (floating feature)

[+F]

e. None to one (featureless segment)

x

The only relationship of these that is possible in conventional segmental theories is that in (1a). The other relationships have been motivated by phonological phenomena in which a particular feature behaves independently of other features or segments. Although the independence of features and segments was originally demonstrated by tonal phenomena, it has also been evident in other nontonal phenomena as will be seen below (see especially the discussion of feature geometry).

One of the tonal phenomena motivating autosegmental representations is the existence and behavior of contour tones in some languages. Rising tones [ǎ] and falling tones [â] are examples of contour tones and are distinguished from level tones, that is, high tones [á] and low tones [à]. Within conventional segmental theories, each of these tones requires a different feature such as [+rising tone] or [+high tone]. Alternatively, within autosegmental phonology, contour tones can be derived from a linear sequence of two different level tones, both of which are associated with the same vowel. A rising tone, then, would be represented as a sequence of a low followed by a high, and a falling tone as a high followed by a low as depicted in (2).

(2)   Autosegmental representation of contour tones

a. Rising tone

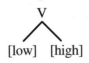

[low]   [high]

b. Falling tone

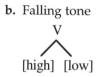

[high] [low]

The derived character of contour tones within autosegmental phonology allows the inventory of tonal features to be kept to a minimum, limited to level tones.

Contour tones also exhibit the phonological behavior of a linear sequence of two level tones. For example, in a language such as Margi, a tonal dissimilation phenomenon occurs such that a prefix and suffix exhibit the opposite tone of a stem. Thus, if the stem has a high tone, as in (3a), the prefix and suffix will have a low tone. Likewise, if the stem has a low tone, as in (3b), the prefix and suffix will have a high tone. The crucial evidence relates to stems with a rising tone, such as that in (3c). In this case, the prefix is realized with a high tone, but the suffix is realized with a low tone.

(3)   Tone dissimilation in Margi (Kenstowicz, 1994)

   a. à tsú gù   "you beat"
   b. á ghà gú   "you reach"
   c. á vĕl gù   "you fly"

The problem for conventional segmental theories is: Why should the opposite of a rising tone be a high tone to the left and a low tone to the right? A natural and unified explanation is offered within autosegmental theory. That is, because a rising tone is at its left edge represented as a level low tone, the opposite tone to the left would be high. Also, because a rising tone is at its right edge represented as a level high tone, the opposite tone to its right would be low. Thus, dissimilation receives a unified account whether the triggering tone is level or contour. Effects of this sort have been termed **edge effects** and constitute evidence for a temporal sequencing of features associated with a single segment as represented in (1c) and (2). Affricates and prenasalized stops are two other classes of sounds that have exhibited edge effects and have been represented as a linear sequence of features associated with one segment.

Tone stability is another phenomenon that has motivated autosegmental representations. More specifically, in a number of tone languages, vowels delete under certain well-defined circumstances, but the tone of the deleted vowel is preserved and reassociates to an adjacent vowel. For example, vowel sequences are prohibited in Margi. However, as a result of certain morphological operations, such sequences would arise but must be resolved phonetically. One of the vowels is deleted but the tone of the deleted vowel is manifest in the preceding or following vowel. The forms in (4) illustrate the delinking (or deletion) of the vowel features from the segmental tier and the stranding of the tonal feature. The stranded tone must be associated with some vowel and thus reassociates with a vowel to the left, resulting in a contour tone.

(4) Tone stability in Margi (Kenstowicz, 1994)

    a. tóró + árĭ → tórórĭ   "threepence"
    b. cédè + árĭ → cédĕrĭ   "money"
    c. fà + árĭ → fărĭ   "farm"
    d. ʃèré + árĭ → ʃèrérĭ   "court"

The independence of tonal features from other segmental features is further evidenced by tonal melodies in various languages. Words of a particular class may exhibit a variety of superficially different tonal patterns depending on the number of syllables in each word. For example, as can be seen in (5) for Mende, a one-syllable word exhibits a rising tone (5a), a two-syllable word exhibits a low tone followed by a high tone (5b), and a three-syllable word exhibits a low tone followed by two high tones (5c). Within conventional segmental theory, each pattern must be represented differently, with no commonalities or explanation for the variation.

(5) Tonal melody in Mende (Leben, 1973)

    a. mbă   "rice"
    b. fàndé   "cotton"
    c. ndàvúlá "sling"

A simple and unified account of these superficial differences is provided if tone is represented on a separate autonomous tier and one tonal melody, namely low-high, is postulated for this particular class of words. Assuming a particular version of the **universal association convention**, the tonal tier can be related to the segmental tier by associating each tone to each vowel as illustrated in (6). In the case of a one-syllable word, all the tones are associated with the only available vowel, yielding a rising tone. In the case of a two-syllable word, the vowel of the first syllable would be associated with a low tone and the vowel of the second syllable with a high tone, yielding level tones on both syllables. In a three-syllable word, as every tone must be associated with at least one vowel in a left-to-right fashion and as every vowel must be associated with at least one tone, the tones would be associated just as in a two-syllable word. The difference is that the final high tone of the melody would be associated with both vowels of the last two syllables.

(6)   Autosegmental representation of a tonal melody

a.

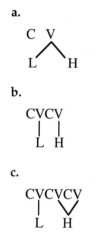

b.

CVCV
│ │
L H

c.

CVCVCV
│ \\/
L   H

The autosegmental representation of tone is also motivated by the differential behavior of morphemes in a language like Margi where, for example, some morphemes take on the tone of an adjacent morpheme, with other morphemes not assimilating. The forms in (7a) exemplify tonal variation in verb stems in accord with the tone of the suffix. The verb stems in (7b), however, do not alternate and are thus resistant to assimilation.

(7)   Margi tone assimilation and nonassimilation (Pulleyblank, 1986)

a. Assimilation

| hù | hó-bá | "take" |
| fà | fá-ŋgə́rí | "take many" |

b. Nonassimilation

| ghà | ghà-bá | ghà-ŋgə́rí | "reach" |
| cú̩ | cí-bá | cí-ŋgə́rí | "speak" |

This phenomenon is readily accounted for if some morphemes, namely the verb stems in (7a), are represented with segmental features alone, without an underlying tone, with other morphemes (the verb stems in [7b]) represented with an underlying tonal feature along with segmen-

tal features. Because the stem morpheme in (7a) is assumed to be toneless underlyingly, the underlying tone of the suffix is free to associate
with both the stem vowel and the suffix, yielding the effect of assimilation. But, the multiple linking of a single tonal feature is prohibited in
(7b), because the verb stem and the suffix are each postulated to already
have different underlying tonal features. This account is schematized in
(8). A dashed line indicates that a feature has spread to the associated
segment.[1]

(8)   Autosegmental representation of tonal (non)assimilation

    a. Spreading of underlying tone to toneless morpheme

    fa + ŋgəri

         H

    b. Nonassimilation

    gha + ba

      L H

This differential representation of morphemes afforded by autosegmental phonology has the empirical consequence that toneless morphemes
can be expected to undergo (i.e., be the target of) tonal assimilations but
not be the trigger of assimilation. Conversely, morphemes with both an
underlying tone and other segmental features can be expected to trigger
assimilation. No such asymmetries would be expected in a segment-
based theory, as features and segments are inseparable.

    Similar asymmetries also obtain if some features or even whole
morphemes are postulated to be segmentless, that is, constituted by a
feature alone with no other segmental properties, as depicted in (1d).
Because the segmental tier is missing in such a case, the postulated feature is said to be **floating**. The presence of a floating feature can only be
detected if it conditions other features on the same tier or if it finds

---

[1]For expository purposes, the tone of the suffix is being depicted as spreading leftward to
the toneless stem. Technically, however, the tone of the suffix would first be associated
with the stem by the universal association convention, with subsequent spreading by rule
to the suffix.

something on the segmental tier to which it can associate. In the latter case, the segmental content would be expected to vary, but the floating feature would be invariant. For example, in Ga'anda, in grammatical constructions involving two nouns, the associative morpheme is realized solely by a high tone on the first vowel of the second noun, independent of the segmental or tonal properties of the nouns, as illustrated in (9).

(9)   Ga'anda associative constructions (Ma Newman, 1971)

    a. āl[2]   "bone"
    b. cùnèwà   "elephant"
    c. āl cúnèwà "bone of elephant"

If the associative morpheme is postulated to be a floating high tone between the two nouns, it can then be associated by rule with the first available vowel of the second noun, explaining both the variable and invariant phonological properties of the grammatical construction.

Finally, it should be noted that segment-based theories have, with difficulty, provided accounts of such phenomena, but these accounts have at best served only to restate the facts. There is nothing about a segment-based representation that should yield these particular effects. The independent behavior of tonal features and segmental features has motivated phonological representations constituted by two autonomous tiers of features, namely a tonal tier and a segmental tier. Similar effects have subsequently been observed for other features, suggesting the need for additional tiers of features and a more elaborate theory of how the various tiers are interrelated. The next section considers such a theory.

Feature Geometry

A general class of theories known as **feature geometry** has adopted the basic insight of autosegmental phonology by postulating tiered representations of features, and has extended the theory by adding a number of other feature tiers and organizing them into a hierarchically structured representation. The hierarchical structuring is intended to explain why some features (but not others) affect or are affected by phonological rules of assimilation (spreading) or neutralization (delinking). The

---

[2]A bar over the vowel designates a level mid tone, which is presumed to be intermediate between level high and low tones.

display in (10) presents a generic version of feature geometry adapted from several different proposals (e.g., Clements, 1985; Paradis & Prunet, 1991; Sagey, 1986).

(10)   A generic feature geometry

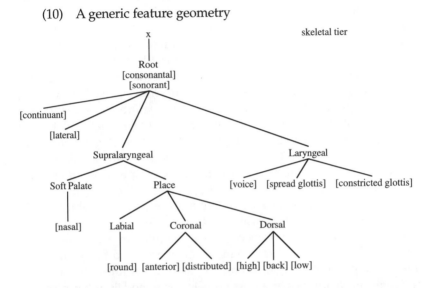

Such geometries entail an elaborate internal structure for segments and can be interpreted as: The highest level of organization depicted is the skeletal tier (designated as x). The skeletal tier represents a timing slot, or a position in a phonological word, to which the content of a phoneme is associated and serves as an interface between prosodic structure and phonemic structure. The root node corresponds with the phoneme and is specifically constituted by the two major class features [consonantal] and [sonorant]. If one root node is associated with two timing slots, the segment is interpreted as long or geminate. On the other hand, if two root nodes are associated with one timing slot on the skeletal tier, a contour segment or diphthong results. The other features of a phoneme are considered dependents of the root node, but are organized into a number of different tiers. The features [continuant] and [lateral] are each represented on separate tiers and are immediately dominated by the root node. The laryngeal features [voice], [spread glottis] and [constricted glottis] are also represented on separate tiers, but they are grouped together under an organizing class node, laryngeal, which is itself immediately dominated by the root node. Yet another organizing class node immediately dominated by the root node is the supralaryngeal node. The supralaryngeal node dominates two other groups of features, namely soft palate and place. The soft palate node has as its dependent the feature [nasal]. The place node groups together all the place of articulation features, each of which is represented on a different tier under the place node. The three different monovalent place of articulation features are labial, coronal and dorsal. Each of these features has a unique set of features as dependents. That is, the feature [round] is associated exclusively with labial, the features [anterior] and [distributed] with coronal, and the features [high], [back] and [low] with dorsal.

A variety of substantively different geometries have thus far been proposed, each of which makes different empirical claims. For example, in geometries like those in (10) where the feature [continuant] is a dependent of the root node, the empirical claim is that that feature should be able to spread or delink as a result of a phonological rule without affecting any other features. Likewise, that feature should remain unaffected by phonological rules that delink or spread features other than the root node. In other geometries, however, the feature [continuant] has been argued to be a dependent of the place node, which would claim that any rule affecting place would also affect [continuant], but not vice versa. Under such a proposal, place assimilation would also effectively be blocked by an intervening segment specified for [continuant] due to the prohibition against crossing association lines. Additionally, although supralaryngeal is a class node in some models, it has no status in others. The crucial evidence relates to whether place features function together with some other group of features in a phonological operation. The essential claim of any geometric structuring of features is that a dependent feature or subordinate node can be operated on independent of higher order features or nodes, but operations defined on a higher order node affect all dependents of that node. Thus, if a rule spreads or delinks the root node, all of the subordinate structures would also be affected. Also, if two or more features are all affected by a single phonological operation, those features must be dominated by the same node. This means, for example, that we might expect to find an empirically motivated assimilation rule that spreads one or all of the laryngeal features but not just two of them. Although debate continues over various aspects of feature geometry, the need for some hierarchical organization of features seems clear.

Among those class nodes that appear to be most well supported are place and laryngeal. The highly common phenomenon in the languages of the world whereby a nasal takes on the place of articulation of a following obstruent supports the spreading of a place node from the obstruent to the preceding nasal, as sketched in (11). Only relevant structure is indicated.

(11)   Place spreading in nasal assimilation

    a. Labial nasal before labial obstruent

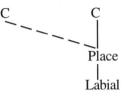

    b. Coronal nasal before a coronal obstruent

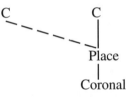

    c. Velar nasal before a velar obstruent

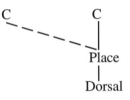

Under this account, there is no need to make reference to any of the specific features of place of articulation, as they all share the higher order class node of place. Thus, a single rule can be formulated that simply spreads place and a fortiori all of its dependent features from an obstruent to an adjacent nasal. The effect of assimilation is achieved by having one place node associated with two different segments.

    Similar assimilatory effects have been observed with laryngeal features, motivating a laryngeal class node. For example, in Classical Greek, the voicing and aspiration contrasts in obstruents are neutralized by an assimilatory process in which stem-final obstruents take on all of the laryngeal features of the immediately following obstruent of the suffix, as exemplified in (12).

(12)   Classical Greek laryngeal assimilation (Kenstowicz, 1994)

      a. trīb-ō   tetrīp-tai   "rub"
      b. grapʰ-ō   gɛgrap-tai   "write"
      c. pɛmp-ō   ɛpɛmpʰ-tʰēn   "send"

    d. trĭb-ō   etrĭpʰ-tʰēn   "rub"
    e. klɛpt-ō   klɛb-dēn   "steal"
    f. grapʰ-ō   grab-dēn   "write"

      Given that all the laryngeal features participate in the assimilation, they must be grouped together under the laryngeal node. The laryngeal node of the suffixal consonant can then spread to the root node of the preceding consonant, and the original laryngeal node of the stem-final consonant is delinked, as illustrated in (13a). Delinking is indicated by drawing two short horizontal lines through an association line. Delinking is necessary to account for the loss of the laryngeal contrasts in this context. This spreading and delinking results in two adjacent obstruents being associated with one and only one laryngeal node (13b).

    (13)   Assimilatory neutralization

        a. Spreading and delinking of laryngeal node

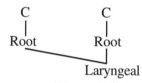

        b. Result of assimilation

          C   C
          | |
       Root   Root
                   |
            Laryngeal

      Support for geometric structure also derives from nonassimilatory phenomena involving reduction or weakening. The idea is that some phonological rules simply delink from the geometric structure one feature or a group of features, resulting in a reduced structure. If a group of features were to be delinked, they would all be required to be dependents of a higher order class node, and it would be the class node that would be delinked. For example, [h] and [ʔ] are often considered reduced variants of /s/ and /t/ (e.g., Durand, 1987; Lass, 1976). They are reduced in the sense that they lack any supralaryngeal articulation. Thus, if a phonological rule were formulated to delink the supralaryngeal node from a structure representing /s/ as in (14a), the resultant structure (14b) would be interpreted as [h]. Weakening of precisely this sort appears to be involved in the aspiration of /s/ in various Caribbean dialects of Spanish (e.g., Harris, 1983).

(14) Weakening

    a. Delinking of supralaryngeal from /s/

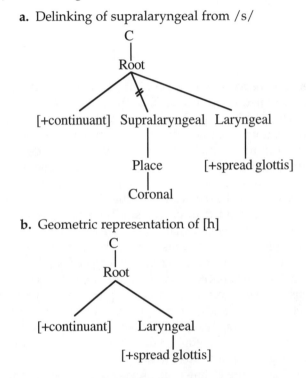

    b. Geometric representation of [h]

The advantage of a geometric account of these and other phenomena is that it, in large part, explains why a rule has the particular result that it does. That is, by limiting a phonological operation (spreading or delinking) to a single terminal feature or to a single node in the geometry, a very specific set of outcomes is predicted. No such constraint is available in nongeometric frameworks since there is no segment-internal organization of features that could serve as the basis to limit the number or types of features involved in a rule. Feature geometry alone does not, however, explain certain other observed asymmetries and transparency effects associated with many phonological rules. For example, certain (classes of) sounds appear to be especially vulnerable to assimilation, with certain other sounds tending to condition assimilations. Additionally, certain sounds appear to be transparent to assimilation, that is, they do not condition or block assimilation. Likewise, certain other sounds appear to be opaque in the sense that they block assimilation. The next section considers a set of theoretical proposals that has been advanced to deal with these issues by differentiating phonological representations in terms of their degree of underlying feature specification.

Underspecification Theory

Early generative theory (Chomsky & Halle, 1968) assumed that phonological rules operated on fully specified representations that included + and − values for each feature. The innovation of underspecification theory has been that not all features can or should be specified underlyingly. That is, some features are absent or underspecified. The idea is that if a feature is not specified at the underlying level, it should not be available to trigger or block any phonological rule. It is these differences in specification that are presumed to coincide with the observed asymmetries and transparency effects alluded to previously. The underspecified features are ultimately filled in (generally late in the derivation) by rules that supply the missing features as defaults. Although different proposals have been advanced about which features are underspecified, there is general agreement that at least noncontrastive features are not specified. Feature specifications for allophonic and redundant properties of pronunciation are thus excluded from underlying representations and not filled in until late in the derivation. For example, then, as nasals in most languages are predictably voiced, the feature [+voice] would be claimed to be absent in the underlying representation of nasals (cf. Rice, 1993 for an alternative perspective). The feature is, however, often contrastive in obstruents and thus cannot be completely underspecified in that class of sounds. The presence versus absence of the voice feature in obstruents and nasals would predict a difference in how these two classes of sounds might condition, for example, voicing in obstruents. (See especially the discussion below of rendaku and Lyman's law in Japanese.)

Proposals differ over the necessity of specifying all contrastive features. Within the framework of contrastive specification (e.g., Steriade, 1987), all contrastive features must be specified. Thus, if the feature [voice] were contrastive in obstruents in some language, both the + and − values of the feature would have to be specified for those pairs of obstruents that do in fact contrast by that feature; but no other sounds would be specified for the feature [voice]. Alternatively, within the framework of radical underspecification (e.g., Archangeli, 1988), generally only marked properties of contrastive features are specified. The unmarked or default value of a contrastive feature must be underspecified, along with all other noncontrastive features. In the case of contrastive voicing, then, only the [+voice] value would be specified for obstruents. The [-voice] property of obstruents and the [+voice] property of nasals would both be underspecified and only later filled in by rule. Under this latter proposal, a noncontrastive feature and the unmarked value of a contrastive feature should act the same phonologically. This prediction is borne out and illustrated in the interaction of rendaku and Lyman's law in Japanese (Mester & Itô, 1989). More specifically, voicing in Japanese is contrastive in obstruents but not in sonorants. The rendaku process voices the initial obstruent of the second member of a compound, as exemplified in (15a). Lyman's law is a separate process that appears to undo rendaku by devoicing the obstruent if a voiced obstruent follows anywhere in the word (15b). The underspecified character of [+voice] as a noncontrastive feature of nasals is supported by the fact that a following nasal (even though phonetically [+voice]) does not trigger Lyman's law (15c). The results of rendaku are thus unaffected by a following nasal. In addition, the underspecified character of [−voice] as the unmarked value of a contrastive feature in obstruents is supported by the fact that an intervening voiceless obstruent does not block Lyman's law (15d). If [−voice] were present in the underlying representation of the intervening voiceless obstruent, the triggering [+voice] feature of the voiced obstruent would not be adjacent to the intended target on the laryngeal tier and should block Lyman's law from applying. The fact is, however, that Lyman's law must be permitted to operate in such cases. By underspecifying [−voice] in obstruents, the [+voice] feature of the trigger and target are adjacent on the laryngeal tier, thus allowing Lyman's law to apply even though many different segments may intervene. The [voice] feature of nasals and voiceless obstruents thus appears to be transparent with respect to Lyman's law and should be underspecified.

(15) Rendaku and Lyman's law in Japanese (Mester & Itô, 1989)

    a. Simple rendaku forms

onna + kokoro	→	onnagokoro
woman heart		"feminine feelings"
neko + ʃita	→	nekodʒita
cat tongue		"aversion to hot food"
eda + ke	→	edage
branch hair		"split hair"

b. Simple Lyman's law forms

kita + kaze   →   kitakaze (*kitagaze)
north wind   "freezing (north) wind"

hana + kazari   →   hanakazari (*hanagazari)
flower decoration   "flower decoration"

c. Forms that do not trigger Lyman's law

ori + kami   →   origami
fold paper   "origami paper"

mizu + seme   →   mizuzeme
water   torture   "water torture"

d. Intervening voiceless segments that do not block Lyman's law

onna + kotoba   →   onnakotoba (*onnagotoba)
woman words   "feminine speech"

doku + tokage   →   dokutokage (*dokudokage)
poison lizard   "Gila monster"

In addition to the transparency effects that obtain by underspecifying features and filling them in late in the derivation, underspecification offers an explanation for certain other asymmetries. For example, by underspecifying certain values of contrastive features (as required under radical underspecification theory), an explanation is offered for why nonassimilatory neutralization rules have the particular product they do. That is, although it is logically possible to achieve the merger of a contrast from a rule that produces any one member of an opposition, it is striking that such rules generally yield only the unmarked member of the contrast (e.g., Houlihan & Iverson, 1979). The highly common phenomenon of word-final devoicing evident in many languages (e.g., German, Catalan, Polish) is an instance of this. Frameworks that treat all features as equal and that account for neutralizations by feature-changing rules have no reason to expect in this instance a devoicing rule like that in (16a) over the unattested (or at least uncommon) rule of word-final voicing (16b).

(16)   Logically possible neutralization rules affecting [voice]

   a. Word-final devoicing

   $[-\text{sonorant}] \rightarrow [-\text{voice}] / \_\_\_\_\_ \#$

   b. Word-final voicing

   [−sonorant] → [+voice] / _____ #

Both rule types are equally complex and would involve the same feature-changing mechanism. Within underspecification theory, however, the attested (and only the attested) neutralization of a voice contrast obtains by delinking the specified laryngeal feature [+voice] from a structure like that in (17a). The resultant structure (17b) is a bare or underspecified laryngeal node. As underspecified features are independently filled in by default, the appropriate [−voice] feature is supplied with no special stipulations (17c).

   (17)   Neutralization by delinking

      a. Specified laryngeal feature

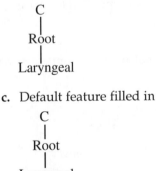

      b. Delinked (underspecified) structure

      c. Default feature filled in

The asymmetric result of nonassimilatory neutralizations thus derives from the delinking of a specified feature with underspecified features filled in by default. Other nonassimilatory neutralizations involving the merger of a manner contrast or of a place contrast would be achieved in the same way. That is, assuming that fricatives are marked relative to stops, fricatives would be specified underlyingly as [+continuant], and stops would be underspecified with the [−continuant] value filled in by default. A neutralization rule delinking [+continuant] would thus result in a stop by default. As only marked values can be specified underlyingly, it would be impossible for a delinking process to derive a fricative from a stop. With regard to place contrasts, it has been argued that coronal is the unmarked place of articulation and is thus underspecified (Paradis & Prunet, 1991). A neutralization rule delinking any of the dependents of place should result in a coronal by default.

Assimilatory phenomena also exhibit asymmetries that receive a natural account within radical underspecification theory. More specifically, unmarked features tend to give way to marked features in assimilations. Precisely this result is expected in underspecification theory if the underspecified character of unmarked features renders them especially vulnerable to being the target of an assimilatory process that spreads a specified (or marked) feature to a segment that is underspecified for that feature. For example, in some languages (e.g., Catalan), only the coronal nasals take on the place of articulation of a following consonant; labial nasals do not assimilate. If coronals are underspecified for place, they are free to acquire a specified place feature (labial or dorsal) by a process that spreads the place node leftward from an adjacent consonant as illustrated in (18a).[3] The resistance of labial nasals to being a target of such a spreading process follows from their already being specified for place (18b).

(18)   Assimilation asymmetries

     a. Underspecified coronal nasals assimilate specified place features

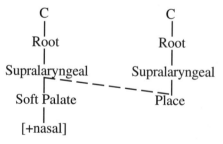

---

[3]As coronals are assumed to be underspecified for place, the place node of coronals would have no dependents and would itself not need to be specified. Under this account of assimilation, it is the place node of the obstruent that spreads to the supralaryngeal node of the preceding nasal and is shared by both segments. A nasal consonant without a place node and not in the context for assimilation would have place and its dependent coronal filled in by default. An alternate view would be to represent coronals with a bare place node, which would serve as the target of an assimilation process that spreads specified terminal place features.

b. Labial nasals do not assimilate

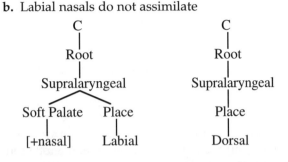

In sum, underspecification theory postulates minimally specified representations, offering an explanation for various observed asymmetries and transparency effects. Those features that are claimed to be specified underlyingly can trigger or block phonological rules, although underspecified features cannot. In addition, the asymmetric result of nonassimilatory neutralization rules follows directly from the delinking of specified features (where only marked contrastive features are specified underlyingly and the unmarked value of contrastive features is filled in by default). Research is continuing in an effort to determine precisely which features must and must not be specified. For a critical review of underspecification theories, see Mohanan (1991). Evidence relevant to particular proposals about the (under)specification of features as well as about the other theoretical frameworks considered here has been drawn almost exclusively from phenomena in fully developed languages. Surprisingly, little attention has been given to phenomena in developing systems (normal or disordered) for the role that they might play in supporting, refuting or modifying any of the proposals sketched above. The remainder of this chapter will attempt to illustrate the value of these newer frameworks for developing systems, as well as the reciprocal value of developing systems for the evaluation of theoretical proposals.

IMPLICATIONS FOR ACQUISITION AND DISORDERS

The rather different concept of phonological structure and representations offered by these nonsegmental frameworks provides some new insights into some long standing problems in the characterization of developing systems. Additionally, in the special case of phonological disorders, these frameworks suggest a rather different focus for clinical treatment with interesting consequences for the projection of children's learning patterns. In the following sections, a broad range of error patterns and acquisition phenomena from children with normal development or with phonological disorders is considered in terms of under-specification theory and feature geometry.

Simple (Nonassimilatory) Substitution Errors

A couple of common error patterns from developing systems will help to illustrate the type of account that is available within underspecification theory as distinct from earlier accounts. One error pattern results in the substitution of alveolars for target velars, and another in the substitution of stops for target fricatives. Both of these patterns are exemplified in the data in (19), from a child with a phonological disorder, Subject 40 (age 6;8).[4]

(19)   Subject 40 (age 6;8)

    a. Substitution of alveolars for target velars

tʌp	"cup"	tʌt	"cut"
tom	"comb"	tabɪ	"cob" (dimin.)
bæti	"back" (dimin.)	wɔti	"rock" (dimin.)
dʌt	"duck"	mɛwt	"milk"

    b. Substitution of stops for target fricatives

bɛɾʊ	"feather"	baɪjə	"fire"
bwuɔbo	"beautiful"	bætjum	"vacuum"
bæn	"van"	weɪbi	"waving"
bihaɪb	"beehive"	tʌndʊ	"thunder"
tutɪ	"toothy"	wit	"wreath"
dit	"sink"	dop	"soap"

Earlier segmental frameworks (e.g., Edwards & Shriberg, 1983; Ingram, 1989; Stoel-Gammon & Dunn, 1985) have characterized such errors as deriving from fully intact adultlike underlying representations. These representations are then systematically converted into the erred outputs by **natural processes** or rules of absolute neutralization. A process of **velar fronting** would change all velars into alveolars (19a), and another process of **stopping** would change all fricatives into

---

[4]This child and others cited herein (unless otherwise noted) were selected from a large-scale Indiana University archival study of the phonological systems and learning patterns of young children with severe phonological disorders (scoring below the 1st percentile relative to age-matched peers on the *Goldman-Fristoe Test of Articulation* (Goldman & Fristoe, 1986).

stops (19b). One problem with such accounts is that they are highly abstract, lacking empirical support for the specific claims about the child's underlying representations. For example, if a child always produces [t] for target /k/, what system-internal evidence is there that the child represents underlying target /k/s specifically as /k/s as opposed to /t/s or any other possible segments? Even perceptual evidence showing that the child can differentiate [t] from [k] when spoken by others does not necessarily show that the distinction is represented in the same way in the child's system. It may even be that the distinction is entirely irrelevant to the child's linguistic system, representing nothing more than a normal psychophysical response. Additionally, the result of these natural processes is entirely arbitrary. For example, why are velars replaced by alveolars rather than by labials? Why are fricatives replaced by stops rather than by nasals? These nonoccurring error patterns would be equally possible under earlier frameworks because they would derive from the same feature-changing mechanism that derives the occurring patterns. For a fuller consideration of these points and additional arguments against such accounts, see the discussion below on shadow-specification and Dinnsen (1993, in press).

An underspecification account avoids both of these problems. First, concrete underlying representations can be postulated, being consistent with the child's production facts while not contradicting properties of the target system. This is achieved by extending the general requirement that underlying representations are underspecified for those features that do not contrast to the child's system. In this way, the child is not being attributed with knowledge of distinctions that are not otherwise manifested in his or her own speech. Second, the only rules that would be necessary are those that are needed independently to fill in default values of features. In the absence of a phonemic contrast in the child's system and with the subsequent lack of an underlying specification, these rules would fill in default values of features, yielding the observed error patterns. For example, with regard to the error pattern in (19a), the absence of any velar obstruents in the child's phonetic inventory means that there is no place of articulation contrast among nonlabial obstruents. Target velars and alveolars would not be differentiated underlyingly and would thus be underspecified for place. Such a representation for the problematic target velars would include only those features that are common to both alveolars and velars, rendering the underlying representation of target velars compatible with the facts of both the child's system and the target system. Given that coronal is the default place of articulation, that feature would be supplied by rule to any representation that is underspecified for place, including the problematic target velars.

A similar underspecification account is available for the error pattern in (19b). As fricatives do not occur in the child's system, the feature [continuant] is noncontrastive and is thus underspecified for target fricatives (and stops). The default value for this feature has been assumed to be [−continuant] and would be supplied by rule to any structure underspecified for manner. The result is that stops replace fricatives, but not vice versa.

An underspecification account of these phenomena differs in several important respects from earlier accounts. On the one hand, the nature of children's underlying representations is at issue. That is, in contrast to earlier accounts, the underspecification account claims that the child has not yet internalized adultlike underlying representations. For a summary of the evidence supporting such a claim, see Dinnsen (in press), Dinnsen, Barlow, and Morrisette (in press), and Dinnsen and Chin (1993, 1994). Secondly, there is the issue of the independent motivation for the rules. That is, in addition to the arbitrariness of the change in feature values effected by the fronting and stopping rules of earlier accounts, such rules must ultimately be lost or suppressed in the acquisition process. In other words, these rules are denied any role in the grammar of a fully developed sound system and thus lack empirical support in those systems. On the other hand, the feature fill-in rules of an underspecification account supply default features to any underspecified representations at any and all stages of acquisition. In the course of acquisition, then, a child's underspecified underlying representations gradually give way to more specified (marked) representations, bringing the child's system into conformity with the target system. The fill-in rules are effectively prevented from applying to those representations that have changed from being underspecified to being specified. The merger of target distinctions thus ceases for all words that have changed underlyingly, but the fill-in rules continue to supply default features to all remaining underspecified representations. For a fuller consideration of this, see the following discussion of the acquisition of phonemic contrasts and Dinnsen (1996a, 1996b).

Shadow-Specification

The claim of an underspecification account as sketched in the section on substitution errors, namely that the child does not differentiate in any way the erred target sound from its substitute, certainly seems appropriate for some children and/or for early stages of acquisition. It does not, however, accord well with the facts for certain other children. That is, some children appear to phonologically differentiate these sounds despite their phonetic identity. To account for such cases, a modification to underspecification theory has been advanced which allows **shadow-specification**, that is, the specification of a default feature for one target sound along with the underspecification of that same feature for another target sound (Dinnsen, 1993). The distinction between a shadow-specified and an underspecified representation thus introduces a phonological distinction without a phonetic distinction. The motivation for and workings of shadow-specification are next briefly summarized.

The phonological differentiation of phonetically identical segments is observable in three different sources of evidence: perceptual differentiation, across-the-board change, and differential phonological behavior. First, the observation that some children (despite their own errors in production) can differentiate target sounds when spoken by others has variously been taken as evidence that the target distinction has been internalized. The precise nature of the distinction has, however, been an issue of considerable controversy. Some have argued that this motivates a two-lexicon model where a target-like representation is encoded in an input perception lexicon and the (erred) production facts are represented in an output production lexicon (e.g., Menn, 1983). Realization rules similar to the stopping and fronting rules above (with all of their associated problems) would connect the two lexicons. One problem with such a model is the duplication that ensues from having to represent much of the same information twice. Also, the results of perceptual experiments have failed to establish that it is exactly the target distinction that has been internalized. At best, they only show that *some* distinction has been internalized. Some studies have even suggested that children may weight acoustic cues of the target system differently in their own systems (e.g., Nittrouer & Studdert-Kennedy, 1987). Shadow-specification and underspecification address these problems by postulating underlying representations that are consistent with both the perception facts and the production facts within a one-lexicon model. For example, a child who exhibits the error pattern in (19a) but perceptually differentiates target /t/ from target /k/ when spoken by others would be claimed to have the following underlying representations for target /t/ and target /k/, respectively:

(20)   Underlying differentiation of phonetically identical segments

    a. Underspecified representation of target /t/

$$
\begin{array}{c}
\text{C} \\
| \\
\text{Root} \\
| \\
\text{Supralaryngeal}
\end{array}
$$

    b. Shadow-specified representation of target /k/

$$
\begin{array}{c}
\text{C} \\
| \\
\text{Root} \\
| \\
\text{Supralaryngeal} \\
| \\
\text{Place} \\
| \\
\text{Coronal}
\end{array}
$$

This difference in representation accords with the child's judgment that there is some difference in place between the two sounds without attributing to the child knowledge of the otherwise empirically unattested dorsal place. If the child does not accurately perceive the dorsal character of the target sound, but does recognize that there is some place distinction, the child can then select as a candidate for specification the default feature for place, coronal. Although this phonological difference is sufficient to yield the desired perceptual result, it also remains consistent with the child's own production facts. That is, nothing is being attributed to the child other than what occurs in the child's system. The phonetic interpretation of the two structures in (20) is the same because a fill-in rule would supply the default feature coronal to the underspecified structure in (20a), rendering it identical to the structure in (20b). Shadow-specification and underspecification thus achieve an underlying distinction that accords well with a child's ability to perceive differences in target sounds while that child also fails to differentiate those sounds in his or her own speech.

Second, the fact that some children's erred pronunciations can change across-the-board to correct productions without any overgeneralization has also been taken as evidence that the target distinctions had to have been correctly internalized beforehand for the child to have known just which words to change (e.g., Smith, 1973). The problem here is the same as above; that is, the need to distinguish phonetically identical segments can motivate a distinction but not necessarily the target distinction. The situation can be illustrated by again considering the error pattern in (19a), where the target distinction between alveolars and velars has been merged phonetically. If, at some subsequent point in time, all and only the errors associated with target velars changed to velars, it would appear that the child would have had to distinguish underlyingly these phonetically identical segments somehow so that the alveolars corresponding with target velars would change but the alveolars corresponding with target alveolars would not change. The distinction afforded by shadow-specification and underspecification is once again sufficient to trigger the change in just those alveolars corresponding to velars. Prior to the change in pronunciation, the child would have internalized representations like those in (20) for target alveolars and target velars. At that point in time, the phonological distinction would still fail to yield a phonetic distinction. The change in pronunciation would subsequently come about from a rule of sound change (similar to rules of sound change in historical linguistics), which shifts one feature specification to another. The rule in this case would be restricted to segments specified as coronal, shifting that feature to another more innovative place feature, namely dorsal. The only segments that would have carried an underlying specification for coronal and thus the only segments that could undergo the rule would be the target velars. The target alveolars would properly be prevented from undergoing the sound change because they lack a specification for place (i.e., they remain underspecified until late in the derivation) and thus do not meet the structural description of the rule.

The third source of evidence that some children phonologically differentiate segments despite their phonetic identity can be seen in the differential behavior of these segments when affected by phonological rules. Consider, for example, the data in (21) from a child with a phonological disorder, Subject 27 (age 4;11), who merged phonetically the target distinction between stops and fricatives by substituting a coronal stop for target /θ/.

(21)　Differential behavior of phonetically identical segments (Subject 27, age 4;11)

a.	it	"eat"	iʔən	"eating"
	bæt	"fat"	bæʔi	"fat" (dimin.)
	but	"boot"	buʔi	"boot" (dimin.)

b. tit   "teeth"   titi   "teeth" (dimin.)
  wit   "wreath"   wʳiti   "wreath" (dimin.)
  maut   "mouth"   maudi   "mouth" (dimin.)

Those [t]s that correspond to target /t/ alternate with [ʔ] word medially, although the coronal stops that correspond to target /θ/ do not alternate. For this child, then, there appear to be two different kinds of [t]: one that alternates with [ʔ] and one that does not alternate. Although this differential behavior corresponds with the target distinction between /t/ and /θ/, all that can be concluded is that the child has internalized *some* distinction (but not necessarily the *target* distinction) and that a phonological rule is sensitive to this distinction. If those [t]s corresponding to target /t/s are underspecified for manner (and place) and those coronal stops corresponding to target /θ/s are shadow-specified for manner (i.e., specified for the default feature [−continuant]) as in (22), then a phonological distinction would be introduced that could condition a rule without also introducing into the child's system segment types that do not otherwise occur.

(22)   Differential representation of phonetically identical segments

    a. Underspecified representation of target /t/

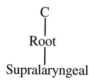

    b. Shadow-specified representation of target /θ/

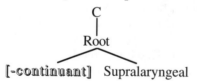

The distinct but substantially underspecified character of target /t/s (22a) would seem to render them especially vulnerable to a weakening process such as glottalization. The simple delinking of supralaryngeal from an already reduced (underspecified) structure would yield a representation that would be interpreted as [ʔ]. The [−continuant] shadow-specification for target fricatives (22b) appears to provide sufficient specificity to the representation of substitute [t]s to distinguish them from target /t/s and insulate them from weakening. Shadow-specification in conjunction with underspecification thus yields the minimally necessary underlying distinction which is sufficient to account for the differential sensitivity of a phonological rule to two segment types that are phonetically identical. The distinction is moreover achieved in terms of phonetically interpretable (nondiacritic) properties that are entirely consistent with the production facts. Similar cases compatible with a shadow-specification account have been reported for other children with phonological disorders (e.g., Anttonen, 1993; Dinnsen, 1995; Dinnsen et al., in press; Fey, 1989; Gierut, 1985: pp. 110–111; Maxwell, 1979) and for normal development (e.g., Applegate, 1961; Smith, 1973).

Assimilatory Substitution Errors

The substitution errors considered previously all involved a marked target sound being replaced by an unmarked sound. Given that marked sounds are often considered more difficult in some sense, their replacement with unmarked or less difficult sounds should not be surprising. There are, however, several other common error patterns that seem to involve just the opposite pattern, namely the substitution of a marked sound for an unmarked sound. Three such error patterns are later considered and are shown to follow naturally and characteristically as contextual assimilations when viewed within a framework of feature geometry and underspecification theory.

Consonant Harmony

One class of errors has been characterized as **consonant harmony** whereby an error results from a consonant coming to agree in place of articulation with another consonant in the same word. A typical example of this phenomenon is reported by Ferguson, Peizer, and Weeks (1973) for a normally developing child, Leslie, and is exemplified in (23).

(23)   Leslie (Ferguson et al., 1973)

    a. 0 years; 11 months

        gaga   "doggie"   bæbæ   "patty (-cake)"

    b. 1;5

        gaga   "doggie"   ŋaŋə   "song"

c. 1;5–2;10

bʌpo	"pencil"	bʌbo, babo	"bottle"
babi	"body"	mɨmɨ	"minute"
fɛfɛ	"sweater"	gækum	"raccoon"
gikay	"this kind"		

These data reveal that target coronal consonants, which are presumably unmarked, are produced in error, being replaced by either labial or velar consonants, both of which are relatively marked. In each instance, however, the substitute consonant agrees in place of articulation with a preceding or following consonant. The account of Ferguson et al., which was formulated in early generative terms, derived the error pattern from a rather complicated place assimilation rule that required several seemingly arbitrary stipulations: (1) only coronal consonants can serve as targets of the assimilation, (2) only labials and velars can serve as triggers of the assimilation, and (3) the rule is bidirectional. Within underspecification theory, however, these conditions follow automatically and need not be stipulated. That is, the underspecified character of coronals renders them especially vulnerable as a target (docking site) for a specified place feature (labial or dorsal) that is spread from and shared with another consonant in the word. The direction of spreading is unrestricted; any consonant underspecified for place can serve as a target of spreading, and any consonant specified for place can serve as a trigger. This account is schematized in (24).[5]

(24)   An underspecification account of consonant harmony

   a. Leftward spreading of place

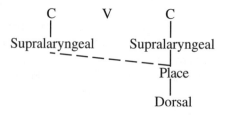

---

[5]The restriction against crossing association lines requires the assumption in these cases that consonants and vowels (or at least their place features) are on separate autosegmental tiers.

b. Rightward spreading of place

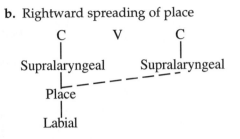

In (24a), an underspecified coronal in word-initial position is serving as the target of place spreading from a postvocalic consonant, which is specified for place (e.g., [gaga] "doggie"). In (24b) an underspecified coronal in postvocalic position is serving as the target of place spreading from a word-initial labial consonant (e.g., [babi] "body").

Similar cases of consonant harmony have been reported for other normally developing children (e.g., Spencer, 1986; Stoel-Gammon & Stemberger, 1994) as well as for children with phonological disorders (e.g., Chin, 1993; Dinnsen, 1995; Dinnsen et al., in press; Gandour, 1981).

Consonant/Vowel Interactions

A different error pattern also occurs such that sometimes (but not always) a marked sound replaces an unmarked sound, but also an unmarked sound replaces a marked sound. Although such an error pattern may appear inconsistent or contradictory, its systematicity is revealed when phonological context is taken into account. An example of such an error pattern is illustrated in (25) with data from a child with a phonological disorder, N.E. (age 4;6) (Williams & Dinnsen, 1987).

(25) N.E. (age 4;6) (Williams & Dinnsen, 1987)

    a. tɛi   "catching"   dɛ   "leg," "dress"

       te   "cage"   de?   "gate"

       tɪkʊ   "chicken"   dɪ   "swim"

       ko   "comb"   go?   "goat"

       ku?   "soup"   guʰ   "tooth"

       ka   "Tom"   ga   "dog"

       kaʰ   "cough"   gʊ   "girl"

b. pɪ   "pinch"   bɪ   "big"
   pʊʰ   "push"   bɛ   "bed"
   piʔ   "peach"   bo   "blow"
   pe   "page"   buʔ   "boot"

The facts in this case are that some (but not all) target coronals are replaced by velars, but also some (but not all) target velars are replaced by coronals. Labial consonants appear to be relatively stable, neither replacing nor being replaced by any other consonant. When the quality of the following vowel is taken into account, it becomes clear that there is no place of articulation contrast among nonlabial consonants. Place of articulation for these consonants appears to be entirely predictable, being conditioned by the quality of the following vowel. Specifically, coronals appear before front vowels, and velars appear before back vowels, independent of the target coronal or dorsal place of articulation. Labial consonants are, however, not conditioned by the following vowel, occurring before both front and back vowels. Place is thus limited to a two-way contrast between labials and nonlabials. An underspecification account of these facts would specify all vowels and only some consonants for place underlyingly. The underspecified consonants would acquire their place features from an assimilatory process that spreads place features from the adjacent vowel.[6] Consonants already specified for place would fail to provide a target for spreading. Given that there is only a two-way contrast in place for consonants, labials would be specified underlyingly for place, and nonlabials (target coronals and dorsals) would be underspecified. This account is schematized in (26).

(26)   Underspecification account of consonant/vowel interactions

   a. Target coronal before a front vowel

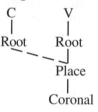

---

[6]A unified feature theory is assumed for consonant and vowel place features (Clements & Hume, 1995).

b. Target coronal before a back vowel

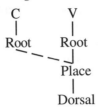

```
  C          V
  |          |
Root       Root
    ‾ ‾ ‾ _|
         Place
          |
        Dorsal
```

c. Target velar before a back vowel

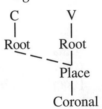

```
  C          V
  |          |
Root       Root
    ‾ ‾ ‾ _|
         Place
          |
        Dorsal
```

d. Target velar before a front vowel

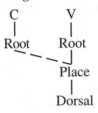

```
  C          V
  |          |
Root       Root
    ‾ ‾ ‾ _|
         Place
          |
        Coronal
```

e. Target labial before a front vowel

```
  C          V
  |          |
Root       Root
  |          |
Place      Place
  |          |
Labial    Coronal
```

This account explains why target coronals and target velars are some-times produced correctly (26a and c) and other times not (26b and d). That is, they appear correctly just in case the target word contains a con-sonant–vowel sequence that agrees in place. Where the target value of the consonant and vowel disagree, an error will result. In the case of

(26e), the specified character of target labial consonants prevents the place feature of the vowel from spreading to the consonant.

Other similar examples of consonant/vowel interactions in normally developing and phonologically disordered systems are presented in terms of feature geometry and underspecification theory in Gierut, Cho and Dinnsen (1993).

Cluster Coalescences

Target consonant clusters are often produced in error by children in the early stages of acquisition. A wide range of errors can occur, but one class is especially relevant to our considerations here. Specifically, some children reduce target clusters to a single consonant where that consonant is not identical to any of the consonants in the target cluster. In these cases, the singleton consonant exhibits some characteristics from each of the consonants of the cluster, hence coalescence. A typical example of coalescence is illustrated in (27) from Joe, a child (age 4;6) with a phonological disorder (Lorentz, 1976).

(27)   Joe (age 4;6) (Lorentz, 1976)

[f]oon	"spoon"	[f]inach	"spinach"
[f]ell	"smell"	[f]ith	"Smith"
[f]amp	"swamp"	[f]oop	"swoop"
[f]ollen	"swollen"		

For this child, the target clusters /sp/, /sm/, and /sw/ are replaced by [f]. The replacement sound bears a striking resemblance to the individual segments of the target cluster, with its continuancy from the first segment and its place of articulation from the second segment. There are, however, other possible replacements that would also bear a resemblance to the individual segments of the cluster, but these seem not to occur. For example, [n] might have replaced /sm/, drawing its place of articulation from the first segment and its manner from the second. In the same fashion, [t] might have replaced /sp/, and [y] might have replaced /sw/. Earlier frameworks have no principled way of distinguishing which features should be able to assimilate in these cases and thus provide the same characterization for both the occurring and the nonoccurring error patterns, predicting that any of these patterns could be expected to occur. An underspecification framework, on the other hand, provides a principled account of these facts. More specifically, the occurring error pattern would involve the spreading of a specified place feature to a segment underspecified for place with the subsequent delinking of the second segment, as depicted in (28).[7] The trigger for coalescence is specified for place and the target is underspecified.

(28)   Underspecification account of coalescence

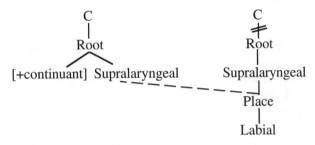

The nonoccurring error pattern is excluded in principle as it would require at the very least the coronal place feature of the first segment, which is underspecified, to be a trigger of place spreading and the second segment to be the target of spreading, although the second segment is already specified for place.

For additional examples and a fuller discussion of cluster coalescence within underspecification and feature geometry, see Chin (1993) and Chin and Dinnsen (1991, 1992).

Reduction Errors

A fourth class of errors introduces the occurrence of a phonological alternation that does not appear to involve a problem with the underlying representation, nor does it appear to have a basis in assimilation. These errors are instead the result of a contextually conditioned reduction process. A typical example of such an error pattern is presented in (29) from a child with a phonological disorder, Subject 35 (age 5;1).

---

[7]The delinking of the second segment is apparently a separate (and possibly optional) process since for some children the target /sw/ clusters are variously realized as [f] and [fw]. Delinking below the C is shown here only for expository purposes. The C-slot would in fact be delinked from a higher order syllable onset.

(29) Subject 35 (age 5;1)

baɪrɪŋ	"biting"	baɪʔ	"bite"
kʌrɪŋ	"cutting"	kʌʔ	"cut"
irɪŋ	"eating"	iʔ	"eat"

These data exhibit an alternation between a word-medial coronal stop and a word-final [ʔ], similar to the error pattern in (21). The occurrence of a coronal stop in word-medial contexts provides some evidence that the child has internalized the correct underlying representations for these words. Earlier frameworks would account for the alternation by a rule that changed the various features of a word-final coronal stop to yield a glottal stop. The problem is, however, that no explanation is offered for the particular effect of the rule. That is, why should the result be a glottal stop rather than a nasal or a fricative? Within a feature geometry framework, precisely the expected result obtains from the simple delinking of the supralaryngeal node in word-final position.

For additional cases of reduction errors derived from delinking processes, see Chin (1993) and Chin and Dinnsen (1991).

Summary of Children's Error Patterns

The above characterizations afforded by underspecification theory and feature geometry suggest that children's errors fall into three general categories differing in the nature of underlying representations. If such a typological characterization is correct, it would be reasonable to expect each of these categories to present a different clinical challenge. For example, the error patterns in (19) and in the section on consonant/vowel interactions were primarily attributed to erroneous (non-target-like) underlying representations. The underlying representations were erroneous in that they lacked many aspects of the required target contrasts. The elimination of such errors would require a child to restructure his or her existing underlying representations through the addition of a new contrast where none existed before. Those error patterns requiring shadow-specification also involved erroneous underlying representations, but erroneous in a different sense. That is, shadow-specified representations reflected an underlying distinction in accord with a target distinction, but the substance of the distinction differed. To eliminate these errors, a child would also have to restructure his or her existing underlying representations, but in this case, one contrastive feature would have to change to another contrastive feature. Finally, errors like those involving consonant harmony, cluster coalescence, and reduction were attributed to essentially adult-like underlying representations that were transformed by phonological rules. Underspecified structures served as targets for these spreading or delinking processes. The elimination of these errors would not require restructuring of underlying representations but would require the child to learn to resist spreading or delinking. These differences in representation constitute testable hypotheses about what a child knows and has yet to learn. At least two questions important to clinical intervention follow from this and warrant further consideration: (1) Are there differences in the relative difficulty of eliminating the different error patterns, and (2) are there differences in the relative efficacy of different forms of treatment for the different error patterns?

ACQUISITION OF PHONEMIC CONTRASTS

A fundamental property of any sound system is the phonemic inventory. Early stages of a developing system exhibit reduced or limited inventories; but ultimate conformity with the target system requires children to add new phonemic contrasts. Phonological theory has long been challenged to provide an adequate characterization of such change. Additionally, children with phonological disorders often require clinical treatment to bring these changes about. The effectiveness of treatment may be enhanced with an improved understanding of phonemic structure and the mechanisms of change. In the following sections, underspecification theory and feature geometry are shown to contribute crucially to a proper characterization of grammar change and to offer insights for the planning of clinical treatment and the projection of learning.

Context-Sensitive Underspecification

The addition of a new contrastive feature to a child's system would appear to require a categorical and instantaneous change in the function of that feature. That is, a feature at any given time in any given context is either contrastive or noncontrastive, and a phoneme is either present or absent in an inventory. The extent of the change may, however, be gradual in that not all words necessarily undergo the change. The theoretical challenge, then, is to arrive at an account that postulates grammar change in accord with the observable changes and that provides a plausible transition from one stage to the next. It has been argued (Dinnsen, 1996a, 1996b; Dinnsen & Chin, 1995) that a particular version of radical underspecification theory, namely **context-sensitive underspecification**, is the only framework capable of providing an adequate account of such facts. In support of this position, an especially revealing set of case studies involving the acquisition of voice, place, and manner contrasts by children with normal or phonologically disordered systems was considered. In each case at an early stage of acquisition, the child lacked a particular target contrast and produced an error pattern that found the target sounds occurring in complementary distribution. At a subsequent stage, the target contrast was introduced, but only in some words, resulting in the persistence of the original error pattern in all other words.

The case of a child with a phonological disorder, A. J. (age 4;11), from Gierut (1986, 1989a) illustrates the issue. Prior to treatment, this child produced only two fricatives, [f] and [s]. While these fricatives normally contrast in English, they occurred in complementary distribution in this child's speech and thus did not contrast. As the data in (30) show, [f] occurred word initially, and [s] occurred elsewhere.

(30)   A. J., age 4;11, Pretreatment (Gierut, 1986, 1989a)

fes	"face"	fu	"food"
faɪn	"vine"	fʌm	"thumb"
fɛm	"them"		
wʊsi	"wolf"	gusi	"goofy"
tisi	"t. v."	wɪs	"with"
gæsi	"glass" (dimin.)	aʊs	"house"

In terms of general underspecification theory, these facts would be accounted for by underspecifying place of articulation for all fricatives since place is noncontrastive and entirely predictable. The values for place would be filled in by an allophonic rule formulated roughly as:

(31)   Given a fricative that is underspecified for place in word-initial position, the default place to be filled in is labial; elsewhere the default place is coronal.

This account and this stage of development are straightforward, being compatible with any version of underspecification theory. The problem arises, however, in the characterization of how development proceeds from this stage. More specifically, a **phonemic split** is needed in order to bring the child's system into conformity with the target system. That is, the allophones [f] and [s], which were associated with a single fricative phoneme in this child's system, would have to reassociate with two different fricative phonemes.

In an effort to induce a phonemic split along these lines, Gierut provided minimal pair contrast treatment, focusing the child's attention on the possible occurrence of [f] postvocalically and [s] word initially. Only moderate success was achieved. That is, following treatment, only a few untreated words were consistently realized with [s] word initially (32a) and only a few others with [f] postvocalically (32b).

(32) A. J. Posttreatment (Gierut, 1986, 1989a)

  a. [s] can occur word initially

sop	"soap"	sɪp	"ship"
sɛo	"shell"		

  b. [f] can occur postvocalically

ifi	"leafy"	pæf	"puff"
lʌf	"love"		

  c. Errors in the occurrence of [f] and [s]

kɔs	"cough"	æsɪŋ	"laughing"
fus	"truth"	fæsɪŋ	"splashing"

Although the words in (32a) and (32b) changed to more closely approximate the target system, the vast majority of words remained unchanged, as illustrated in (32c). The forms in (32c) preserved the earlier pattern of distribution with [f] in initial position and [s] postvocalically. The change was clearly not across-the-board. However, even though only a few words changed, technically a phonemic split was achieved. Both [f] and [s] were used contrastively in word-initial position and in postvocalic position after treatment, although not always appropriately.

The characterization of these changes (as well as the absence of phonetic change) following clinical intervention is problematic for a theory of contrastive specification (and, for many of the same reasons, for frameworks that assume fully specified representations[8]). At the point the phonemic split was effected, all occurrences of [f] and [s] (whether correct or incorrect) would have had to change from being underspecified for place to being contrastively specified. The reason for this is that

[8]For details of how an earlier framework with fully specified representations would account for the two stages, see Gierut (1986).

contrastive specification is determined from the phonemic inventory. If a feature has suddenly become contrastive, then the phonemic inventory has also changed. Also, the rule in (31) would no longer have been necessary since all values for place would be specified underlyingly, resulting in the rule's loss. Thus, even though the phonetic changes did not occur across-the-board, all lexical items with fricatives would have had to restructure in this framework. Although such a characterization certainly seems warranted for those few words where there was a phonetic change (32a and b), an underlying change would also have been required for the many other words that did not change phonetically (32c). That is, the word-initial fricatives that did not change phonetically would have had to change underlyingly from being underspecified for place to being specified as labial. Likewise, the postvocalic fricatives that did not change phonetically would also have had to change underlyingly from being underspecified for place to being specified as coronal. These required changes at the underlying level furthermore would result in many specifications that contradict the facts of the target system. For example, the many phonetically unchanged [f]s in word-initial position that corresponded with target coronals would have had to be specified as labial after treatment. Similarly, the phonetically unchanged [s]s in postvocalic position that corresponded with target labials would have had to be specified as coronal. A contrastive specification framework would claim further that it was purely accidental that fricatives changed underlyingly as they did. For example, why did an underspecified fricative in word-initial position change more often than not at the underlying level to a specified labial? Also, why did underspecified fricatives in postvocalic position change more often than not to a specified coronal? In other words, why did many items change in just that way that preserved the pattern of distribution that had been associated with the original allophonic rule in (31)? The specification of place in this framework would deny any connection with or influence from the rule that had operated in the immediately preceding stage.

These problems are avoided if the particular version of radical underspecification theory already discussed is adopted, namely context-sensitive underspecification. Recall that radical underspecification theory allows only one value of a contrastive feature to be specified underlyingly. Context-sensitive underspecification also allows only one value of a contrastive feature to be specified underlyingly, but this constraint is limited to given contexts. This has the effect of allowing both values of a contrastive feature to be specified underlyingly, but never in the same context. Precisely this effect is what is needed to adequately account for facts of the sort noted. That is, at the point the place of articulation contrast was introduced, both contrastive features, labial and coronal, could be specified underlyingly, but not in the same contexts and not even in all words. In fact, only those words that changed phonetically would change underlyingly. The few postvocalic fricatives that changed phonetically to [f] (32b) would have changed underlyingly from being underspecified to being specified as labial. The many postvocalic fricatives that did not change phonetically (32c) would remain underspecified for place with the default coronal value being filled in by the earlier rule in (31). Although many of these postvocalic fricatives corresponded with target [f], a contradiction in specification would be avoided by their remaining underspecified for place. The seemingly contradictory coronal feature would be supplied by rule. Similarly, the few word-initial fricatives that changed phonetically to [s] (32a) would have changed underlyingly from being underspecified to being specified as coronal. The many other word-initial fricatives that did not change phonetically (32c) would have remained underspecified for place with the default labial feature being filled in by the rule in (31). Some of these corresponded with target [s], but a contradiction with the target specification would be avoided because they would have remained underspecified for place. The consequence is that coronal would be the specified value for fricatives word initially and labial the specified value postvocalically. The rule in (31) would properly be prevented from applying to those forms in (32a) and (32b) because they would have already been specified for place. The rule would apply to all other words that were underspecified for place (32c).

Under the context-sensitive underspecification account, all phonetic changes accorded perfectly with changes in underlying specifications. Also, none of the required underlying specifications contradicted target specifications for place. Finally, continuity was preserved across stages by ascribing minimal change to the system. That is, many representations remained underspecified and the fill-in rule in (31) continued to predict the distribution of place features, accounting for the persistence of the error pattern.

Geometric Cyclicity

It has always been difficult to predict which particular sound(s), if any, will be acquired by a child, even when clinical treatment is provided. The thought is that there is a specifiable order to the acquisition of phonemic contrasts and that some sounds may be easier (in some sense) than others and thus would be acquired before more difficult sounds. It has been tempting in this regard to appeal to developmental norms (e.g., Smit, Hand, Freilinger, Bernthal, & Bird, 1990) as a predictor of the order of acquisition of phonemes, assuming that earlier-acquired sounds are easier than later-acquired sounds. The literature is, however, replete with exceptions where some later-acquired (presumably more difficult) sounds are acquired before some earlier-acquired sounds (e.g., Gierut, Morrisette, Hughes, & Rowland, 1996). If, however, the focus is shifted away from particular sounds to featural distinctions of sounds and moreover to a particular organization of features, a principle emerges. In a series of descriptive and experimental studies (Gierut, 1994a, b; Gierut & Morrisette, 1995; Gierut, Simmerman, & Neumann, 1994), Gierut has identified a principle of phonemic acquisition that crucially appeals to subsegmental structure in accord with the organization of features as prescribed by feature geometry. The principle, **laryngeal-supralaryngeal cyclicity**, maintains that phonemic inventories are expanded over time by adding a feature distinction from either the laryngeal domain of the geometry or the supralaryngeal (place or manner) domain in an alternating sequential fashion. As a result, the principle can account for both the symmetrical and asymmetrical character of phonemic inventories at the various different points in time. For example, consider a possible phonemic inventory like that in (33a) that limits its obstruents to /p b t/. Such an inventory would be judged asymmetrical, lacking a voice distinction in coronals. The subsequent introduction of a voice distinction with /d/ as in (33b) is one possible elaboration of the inventory in (33a) and would render the inventory symmetrical. The subsequent addition of /k/ to the inventory in (33b), representing a new supralaryngeal distinction, is a further possible expansion and would render the new inventory in (33c) asymmetrical again, this time with respect to the absence of a voice distinction in velars. The principle also predicts that certain other logical possibilities for inventory expansion will not occur. More specifically, two distinctions of the same type (i.e., either two laryngeal distinctions or two supralaryngeal distinctions) cannot be added to an inventory in succession. For example, then, /s/ could not be added to the inventory in (33a) immediately after the addition of the supralaryngeal distinction associated with /t/ to yield the inventory in (33d). The reason for this is that /s/ would be introducing a supralaryngeal manner distinction to an inventory that was already rendered asymmetrical from the immediately prior addition of /t/. The principle also excludes the possibility of two different sounds being added to an inventory at the same point in time if one of the sounds elaborates the inventory by a laryngeal distinction and the other sound by a supralaryngeal distinction. For example, both /k/ and /g/ could not be added at the same point in time to the inventory in

(33b) to yield the inventory in (33e). The reason for this is that these two sounds would introduce a supralaryngeal dorsal place distinction as well as a laryngeal voice distinction within the dorsals. This is not to say that two or more sounds cannot be added to an inventory at the same time. In fact, multiple sounds can be added at the same point in time if they all introduce either a supralaryngeal distinction or a laryngeal distinction. For example, /f/ and /s/ could both be added to an inventory like that in (33b) to yield the inventory in (33f) because these sounds introduce only supralaryngeal (place and manner) distinctions; the laryngeal properties of the fricatives would be noncontrastive and thus predictable.

(33)   Logically possible obstruent inventories

   a. Early asymmetrical inventory

   p   t
   b

   b. Symmetrical inventory from expansion of (a)

   p   t
   b   d

   c. Asymmetrical inventory from expansion of (b)

   p   t   k
   b   d

   d. Nonoccurring expansion of (a)

   p   t
   b

         s

   e. Nonoccurring expansion of (b)

   p   t   k
   b   d   g

   f. Permissible expansion of (b)

   p   t
   b   d
   f   s

Any earlier framework lacking a subsegmental organization of features would find it difficult to explain why just certain features (and thus just certain sounds) can be added to an inventory but others cannot. Feature geometry, on the other hand, imposes a grouping of features, where each group not only serves as the constituent domains of phonological rules but also as the constituent domains of a principle that allows inventories to expand by elaborating features in one domain and then in the other domain in an alternating fashion.

Gierut's work has also shown that this principle is exploitable in the planning of treatment and the projection of learning. Consider, for example, a child with an inventory like that in (33a), where a laryngeal distinction would be the next expected distinction to be acquired. At least two different treatment strategies are possible. On the one hand, treatment could focus on introducing that expected laryngeal distinction in-phase by teaching /d/. On the other hand, the expected distinction could be skipped with treatment focusing instead on the next phase of the cycle, namely on introducing another supralaryngeal distinction by teaching /s/. Under this latter approach, the treated sound could not be acquired unless the prerequisite (untreated) laryngeal distinction is acquired beforehand. In a comparison of these two treatment strategies, Gierut found that the latter approach was more efficacious, resulting in more new (untreated) phonemes being added to the children's inventories.

Maximal Opposition Treatment

In another series of descriptive and experimental studies (Gierut, 1989b, 1990, 1991, 1992; Gierut & Neumann, 1992), an especially interesting learning effect has been uncovered that derives from a special type of minimal pair contrast treatment, namely **maximal opposition treatment**. This form of treatment may also find a basis in feature geometry. In conventional minimal pair treatment, a target sound that is produced in error is contrasted with its substitute. Consequently, if a child substitutes [t] for target /k/, as in (19a) above, treatment would expose the child to target words that differ by /t/ and /k/, that is, "top" versus "cop." This form of minimal pair treatment focuses on the minimal difference that obtains between the target sound and its substitute. Alternatively, in maximal opposition treatment, a target sound that is produced in error is contrasted with some other target sound that differs from the erred sound in many features and is uninvolved with the error pattern. Thus, given the same error pattern in (19a), treatment might oppose target words that differ by /k/ versus /m/, that is, "can" versus "man." This form of minimal pair treatment focuses on maximal (rather than minimal) differences between sounds. The magnitude of a difference between minimal pairs can be measured by the number or type of feature differences. In the example of conventional minimal pair treatment noted here, treatment targets would differ only by place of articulation features. In the example of maximal opposition treatment, however, the treatment targets would differ by many more features, including place, voice, manner, and sonorancy. Gierut found that maximal opposition treatment was more effective than conventional minimal pair treatment in inducing the addition of more new phonemes to a child's inventory. This effect was augmented if the maximally opposed minimal pairs differed in at least sonorancy. This effect has no ready explanation in earlier frameworks because all features are equal and undifferentiated. Within feature geometry, however, differences in the number of features and the type of features are directly encoded in the number and relationship of tiers in the geometric structure. The fact, then, that sonorancy is the most important featural difference between sounds to be opposed in treatment follows directly in feature geometry from the fact that sonorancy is a property of the highest-order segmental tier, namely the root node. Additionally, if the opposing sounds also differ in voice, place, and manner features, all the other organizing nodes and tiers of the geometry are also being contrasted. If treatment is viewed as an attempt to reveal new phonemic structure to the child, maximal opposition treatment illuminates or highlights for the child all aspects of the contrasting structures. Conventional minimal pair treatment, on the other hand, selects treatment targets that are the same in all respects, except for one low-level property, namely the presence versus absence of a terminal feature. Maximal opposition treatment seems to exploit the full structure and organization of contrasting sounds in a way that conventional minimal pair treatment cannot. Treatment that appeals to the basic constructs of feature geometry as illustrated offers a principled basis for the selection of treatment targets and an explanation for certain treatment effects, including the order of acquisition of phonemes and the relative efficacy of different treatment methods.

CONCLUSION

The nonsegmental frameworks of autosegmental phonology, feature geometry, and underspecification theory have revolutionized our concepts of phonological structure and representations by postulating minimally specified, multilayered, and hierarchically organized representations. Although these frameworks have been motivated by phenomena in fully developed languages, this chapter has been developed to show that phenomena in developing systems are equally amenable and illuminating. The error patterns found in children's speech reflect the same asymmetries and transparency effects found in fully developed systems. An explanation is thus offered for why particular sounds are produced in error and why the error takes the form it does. Many errors appear to be attributable to the substance of children's underlying representations. When their underlying representations are erroneous due to a lack of differentiation, the underspecified character of these representations renders them especially vulnerable to being produced in error. But even correctly internalized representations that are radically underspecified can also be vulnerable to error. One reason for this is that underspecified representations naturally attract nearby specified features through assimilatory feature-spreading processes. The actual form of errors predictably arises then in many instances from unconstrained spreading. When underspecified representations are not possible targets for assimilation, the form of the error follows predictably from an unmarked feature being filled in by default. Additionally, appeal to underspecification and shadow-specification has allowed us to differentiate these error patterns from certain other superficially similar (but crucially different) errors. That is, some errors are associated with sounds that are typologically marked in the target system, and the form of the error is always unmarked and unaffected by assimilation. Also, despite the fact that these errors result in a phonetic merger of a target contrast, the child evidences some knowledge of an underlying distinction. Precisely this result obtains in cases where a child has internalized underspecified and shadow-specified representations. An underlying distinction is thus introduced in accord with the child's presumed knowledge of a distinction. The distinction is, however, entirely consistent with the child's production facts and does not attribute to the child underlying distinctions that cannot be observed in the child's speech. Because only default features can be shadow-specified, underspecified and shadow-specified representations will have the same phonetic interpretation, resulting in an unmarked sound. The specificity of shadow-specified representations has the further consequence of insulating them from being possible targets of assimilatory feature-spreading processes. An explanation is thus offered for why phonetically identical sounds can act differently in a child's system. Although these nonsegmental frameworks properly differentiate some superficially similar error patterns, they also provide a unified characterization of certain other superficially different error patterns. Recall, for example, that the superficially different "fronting" and "backing" errors in N.E.'s speech (25) were both found to follow from the same underspecification of place with spreading from an adjacent vowel. The characterization and explanation of error patterns that emerge from these nonsegmental frameworks are quite different from earlier accounts and hold promise for new insights into acquisition and treatment. A model of acquisition emerges in which children's underlying representations are largely underspecified in early stages of acquisition. As time goes on, new distinctions are introduced with minimal change to the grammar in a way that respects constraints imposed by context-sensitive underspecification theory. Additionally, phonemic inventories appear to expand in accord with a principle of cyclicity that crucially appeals to subsegmental geometric structure. Treatment designed around such a principle and associated structure has been able to exploit these new insights to yield greater improvements in children's sound systems. As developing systems are reconsidered in light of these nonsegmental frameworks, it is expected that other long standing problems can be resolved and that treatment will continue to take advantage of our improved understanding of these systems. It is also expected that developing systems will play a greater role in the (re)formulation and evaluation of theoretical proposals.

Although the frameworks and issues considered in this chapter have focused primarily on the nature of representations, these representations also have many other important theoretical consequences. In standard derivational theories such as generative phonology and natural phonology, where underlying representations are converted into phonetic representations, the nature of rules (or processes) is severely constrained by these representations. For example, rules are triggered by representations only if those representations are specified for some feature. Also, rules can only spread or delete certain features or groups of features as provided by feature geometry. The nature of representations is also central to constraint-based theories such as optimality theory (e.g., Prince & Smolensky, 1993). In such frameworks, a ranked set of universal constraints selects for any given input (underlying representation) an optimal output from among all possible output candidates. Although constraints are formulated in terms of output properties, these properties must correspond with the input in particular ways and to a particular degree. The only two elements of grammar that can vary are inputs and/or constraint rankings. If input representations could not change over time or across individuals, the acquisition process would be limited to changes in constraint rankings. Greater evidence of across-the-board change might then be expected to occur in the course of phonological development. However, as many aspects of phonological development diffuse gradually through the lexicon, change and variation in the substance of children's underlying representations seems a more likely focal point. For a fuller discussion of the role of representations in constraint-based approaches to acquisition, see Dinnsen and Barlow (1996).

FURTHER READINGS

Carr, P. (1993). *Phonology*. New York: St. Martin's Press.
Goldsmith, J. A. (1990). *Autosegmental phonology and metrical phonology*. Cambridge, MA: Blackwell.
Goldsmith, J. A. (Ed.). (1995). *The handbook of phonological theory*. Cambridge, MA: Blackwell.
Spencer, A. (1996). *Phonology: Theory and description*. Cambridge, MA: Blackwell.

ACKNOWLEDGMENTS

I am especially grateful to Jessica Barlow, Steve Chin, and Judith Gierut for their many helpful comments and discussions on this and related work. This work was supported in part by grants from the National Institutes of Health (DC00260 and DC01694).

REFERENCES

Anttonen, E. C. (1993). *Specification and representation in phonemic acquisition.* Master's thesis, Indiana University, Bloomington.
Applegate, J. R. (1961). Phonological rules of a subdialect of English. *Word, 17,* 186–193.
Archangeli, D. (1988). Aspects of underspecification theory. *Phonology, 5,* 183–207.
Chin, S. B. (1993). *The organization and specification of features in functionally disordered phonologies.* Doctoral dissertation, Indiana University, Bloomington.
Chin, S. B., & Dinnsen, D. A. (1991). Feature geometry in disordered phonologies. *Clinical Linguistics and Phonetics, 5,* 329–337.
Chin, S. B., & Dinnsen, D. A. (1992). Consonant clusters in disordered speech: Constraints and correspondence patterns. *Journal of Child Language, 19,* 259–285.
Chomsky, N., & Halle, M. (1968). *The sound pattern of English.* New York: Harper & Row.
Clements, G. N. (1985). The geometry of phonological features. *Phonology, 2,* 225–252.

Clements, G. N., & Hume, E. V. (1995). The internal organization of speech sounds. In J. A. Goldsmith (Ed.), *The handbook of phonological theory* (pp. 245–306). Cambridge, MA: Blackwell.

Dinnsen, D. A. (1993). Underspecification in phonological disorders. In M. Eid & G. Iverson (Eds.), *Principles and prediction: The analysis of natural language: Papers in honor of Gerald Sanders* (pp. 287–304). Philadelphia: John Benjamins.

Dinnsen, D. A. (1995, November). *The manner node reconsidered*. Paper presented at the 20th Annual Boston University Conference on Language Development, Boston, MA.

Dinnsen, D. A. (1996a). Context effects in the acquisition of fricatives. In B. Bernhardt, D. Ingram, & J. Gilbert (Eds.), *Proceedings of the UBC International Conference on Phonological Acquisition* (pp. 136–148). Somerville, MA: Cascadilla Press.

Dinnsen, D. A. (1996b). Context-sensitive underspecification and the acquisition of phonemic contrasts. *Journal of Child Language, 23,* 57–79.

Dinnsen, D. A. (in press). Some empirical and theoretical issues in disordered child phonology. In T. K. Bhatia & W. C. Ritchie (Eds.), *Handbook on child language acquisition.* New York: Academic Press.

Dinnsen, D. A., & Barlow, J. A. (1996). Chain shifts in acquisition. Under editorial review.

Dinnsen, D. A., Barlow, J. A., & Morrisette, M. L. (in press). Long-distance place assimilation with an interacting error pattern in phonological acquisition. *Clinical Linguistics and Phonetics.*

Dinnsen, D. A., & Chin, S. B. (1993). Individual differences in phonological disorders and implications for a theory of acquisition. In F. R. Eckman (Ed.), *Confluence: Linguistics, L2 acquisition, and speech pathology* (pp. 137–152). Amsterdam: John Benjamins.

Dinnsen, D. A., & Chin, S. B. (1994). Independent and relational accounts of phonological disorders. In M. Yavas (Ed.), *First and second language phonology* (pp. 135–148). San Diego: Singular Publishing Group.

Dinnsen, D. A., & Chin, S. B. (1995). On the natural domain of phonological disorders. In J. Archibald (Ed.), *Phonological acquisition and phonological theory* (pp. 135–150). Hillsdale, NJ: Erlbaum.

Durand, J. (1987). On the phonological status of glides: The evidence from Malay. In J. Anderson & J. Durand (Eds.), *Explorations in dependency phonology* (pp. 79–108). Dordrecht: Foris.

Edwards, M. L., & Shriberg, L. D. (1983). *Phonology: Applications in communicative disorders.* San Diego: College-Hill Press.

Ferguson, C. A., Peizer, D. B., & Weeks, T. E. (1973). Model-and-replica phonological grammar of a child's first words. *Lingua, 31,* 35–65.

Fey, M. E. (1989). Describing developing phonological systems: A response to Gierut. *Applied Psycholinguistics, 10,* 455–467.

Gandour, J. (1981). The nondeviant nature of deviant phonological systems. *Journal of Communication Disorders, 14,* 11–29.

Gierut, J. A. (1985). *On the relationship between phonological knowledge and generalization learning in misarticulating children.* Doctoral dissertation, Indiana University Linguistics Club.

Gierut, J. A. (1986). Sound change: A phonemic split in a misarticulating child. *Applied Psycholinguistics, 7,* 57–68.

Gierut, J. A. (1989a). Developing descriptions of phonological systems: A sur-rebuttal. *Applied Psycholinguistics, 10,* 469–473.

Gierut, J. A. (1989b). Maximal opposition approach to phonological treatment. *Journal of Speech and Hearing Disorders, 54,* 9–19.

Gierut, J. A. (1990). Differential learning of phonological oppositions. *Journal of Speech and Hearing Research, 33,* 540–549.

Gierut, J. A. (1991). Homonymy in phonological change. *Clinical Linguistics and Phonetics, 5,* 119–137.

Gierut, J. A. (1992). The conditions and course of clinically-induced phonological change. *Journal of Speech and Hearing Research, 35,* 1049–1063.

Gierut, J. A. (1994a). Cyclicity in the acquisition of phonemic distinctions. *Lingua, 94,* 1–23.

Gierut, J. A. (1994b). An experimental test of phonemic cyclicity. *Journal of Child Language, 23,* 291–316.

Gierut, J. A., Cho, M.-H., & Dinnsen, D. A. (1993). Geometric accounts of consonant-vowel interactions in developing systems. *Clinical Linguistics and Phonetics, 7,* 219–236.

Gierut, J. A., & Morrisette, M. L. (1995). Triggering a principle of phonemic acquisition. *Clinical Linguistics and Phonetics, 10,* 15–30.

Gierut, J. A., Morrisette, M. L., Hughes, M. T., & Rowland, S. (1996). Phonological treatment efficacy and developmental norms. *Language, Speech, and Hearing Services in Schools, 27,* 215–230.

Gierut, J. A., & Neumann, H. J. (1992). Teaching and learning /θ/: A nonconfound. *Clinical Linguistics and Phonetics, 6,* 191–200.

Gierut, J. A., Simmerman, C. L., & Neumann, H. J. (1994). Phonemic structures of delayed phonological systems. *Journal of Child Language, 21,* 291–316.

Goldman, R., & Fristoe, M. (1986). *Goldman-Fristoe Test of Articulation.* Circle Pines, MN: American Guidance Service.

Goldsmith, J. (1979). *Autosegmental phonology.* New York: Garland.

Harris, J. (1983). *Syllable structure and stress in Spanish.* Cambridge, MA: MIT Press.

Houlihan, K., & Iverson, G. K. (1979). Functionally-constrained phonology. In D. A. Dinnsen (Ed.), *Current approaches to phonological theory* (pp. 50–73). Bloomington: Indiana University Press.

Ingram, D. (1989). *Phonological disability in children* (2nd ed.). San Diego: Singular Publishing Group.

Kenstowicz, M. (1994). *Phonology in generative grammar.* Cambridge, MA: Blackwell.

Lass, R. (1976). *English phonology and phonological theory.* London: Cambridge University Press.

Leben, W. (1973). *Suprasegmental phonology*. Doctoral dissertation, Massachusetts Institute of Technology, Cambridge.

Lorentz, J. P. (1976). An analysis of some deviant phonological rules of English. In D. M. Morehead & A. E. Morehead (Eds.), *Normal and deficient child language* (pp. 29–60). Baltimore: University Park Press.

Ma Newman, R. (1971). Downstep in Ga'anda. *Journal of African Languages, 10,* 15–27.

Maxwell, E. M. (1979). Competing analyses of a deviant phonology. *Glossa, 13,* 181–214.

Menn, L. (1983). Development of articulatory, phonetic, and phonological capabilities. In B. Butterworth (Ed.), *Language production 2: Development, writing and other language processes* (pp. 3–50). New York: Academic Press.

Mester, R. A., & Itô, J. (1989). Feature predictability and underspecification: Palatal prosody in Japanese mimetics. *Language, 65,* 258–293.

Mohanan, K. P. (1991). On the bases of radical underspecification. *Natural Language and Linguistic Theory, 9,* 285–325.

Nittrouer, S., & Studdert-Kennedy, M. (1987). The role of coarticulatory effects in the perception of fricatives by children and adults. *Journal of Speech and Hearing Research, 30,* 319–329.

Paradis, C., & Prunet, J. F. (Eds.). (1991). *Phonetics and phonology: Volume 2: The special status of soronals: Internal and external evidence*. San Diego: Academic Press.

Prince, A., & Smolensky, P. (1993). *Optimality theory: Constraint interaction in generative grammar* (Technical Report No. 2 of the Rutgers Center for Cognitive Science). New Brunswick, NJ: Rutgers University.

Pulleyblank, D. (1986). *Tone in lexical phonology*. Dordrecht: Reidel.

Rice, K. D. (1993). A re-examination of the feature [sonorant]: The status of "sonorant obstruents." *Language, 69,* 308–344.

Sagey, E. C. (1986). *The representation of features and relations in non-linear phonology*. Doctoral dissertation, Massachusetts Institute of Technology, Cambridge.

Smit, A. B., Hand, L., Freilinger, J. J., Bernthal, J. E., & Bird, A. (1990). The Iowa articulation norms project and its Nebraska replication. *Journal of Speech and Hearing Disorders, 55,* 779–798.

Smith, N. V. (1973). *The acquisition of phonology: A case study*. Cambridge, England: Cambridge University Press.

Spencer, A. (1986). Towards a theory of phonological development. *Lingua, 68,* 3–38.

Steriade, D. (1987). Redundant values. *Chicago Linguistic Society, 23,* 339–362.

Stoel-Gammon, C., & Dunn, C. (1985). *Normal and disordered phonology in children*. Austin, TX: PRO-ED.

Stoel-Gammon, C., & Stemberger, J. P. (1994). Consonant harmony and phonological underspecification in child speech. In M. Yavas (Ed.), *First and second language phonology* (pp. 63–80). San Diego: Singular Publishing Group.

Williams, A. L., & Dinnsen, D. A. (1987). A problem of allophonic variation in a speech disordered child. *Innovations in Linguistic Education, 5,* 85–90.

CHAPTER

Monovalent Phonologies: Dependency Phonology and an Introduction to Government Phonology

MARTIN J. BALL

In this chapter, approaches to phonological analysis are examined that operate with unary phonological primes and with some method of relating these primes in a hierarchical fashion. The best developed of these accounts is Dependency Phonology, but some derivatives of the dependency approach are also examined later in the chapter.

Before attending to Dependency Phonology (DP), the purpose of phonological analysis within the clinical context is discussed. We need to know what a phonological analysis is for before we can decide which approach is best for which kind of disorder. In clinical terms, we need a phonological analysis to specify what sound system a particular patient is using, so we can become aware of both the phonetic and phonological (i.e., contrastive) abilities of the speaker.

However, we also need to get explicit information as to how this phonology relates to the target phonology of the speech community within which the patient operates. This last point allows the analysis to feed directly into remediation: An effective phonological analysis informs phonological therapy.

What kind of phonological model can we best use to meet these aims? On the one hand, if the patient's realizations of the target sound system are extremely variable, with little or no patterns or predictable distribution of sounds, then it is arguable that a phonological analysis of any type is not helpful, if indeed possible. On the other, if the patient simply exhibits one or two across-the-board substitutions of a straight-forward type (e.g., alveolar for velar), then it is difficult to argue that any one type of phonological approach would be a great deal better than any other at capturing what is going on. However, such extremes are the exception rather than the norm, and we will usually be faced with situations where a mixture of simple and less simple phonological changes interact within the data. It is in such situations where we may start to look at the contributions of different models of phonological analysis to see which meet best the criteria noted above.

In this chapter, I argue that Dependency Phonology has advantages over other models in the description of disordered speech. I am not, however, asserting that it is the only effective approach, nor that it is superior on all occasions; but I hope to illustrate its positive features in a series of examples of clinical data. First, we will look at the debate concerning the nature of phonological units.

PHONOLOGICAL UNITS

In this section certain aspects of the debate as to what constitute phonological units are examined—in particular, minimal phonological units. Even current proponents of the segment as an important phonological unit (for example, Ohala, 1992) recognize that some kind of subsegmental element is required in an adequate phonological theory. The debate arises in trying to decide what sort of subsegmental element it should be.

Features

As Ohala (1992, p. 166) states, "the segmental or articulated character of speech has been one of the cornerstones of phonology since its beginnings some two-and-a-half millennia ago" (see also Durand, 1990, pp. 12–13 for discussion on this issue). However, as phonologists have long realized, units smaller than the segment can be posited and, indeed, are needed if we want to be able to make statements about natural classes of segments and the phonological processes affecting them. The answer to this problem has normally been some kind of feature, or component, that might be thought of as making up a segment in conjunction with others.[1] Such a feature can then be isolated and serve as the input to a phonological process or as a method of grouping segments together into natural classes and so on.

The notion of the phonological feature as commonly found in modern phonological approaches derives largely from the work of the Prague School of linguistics. However, while Trubetzkoy (1969 [original 1939]) for example, considered a range of feature types, later work by Jakobson, Fant, and Halle (1952), Jakobson and Halle (1956), and Chomsky and Halle (1968) drew on only a subset of these feature types. In particular, they proposed systems of phonological distinctive features that were binary, with alternative unary and scalar features considered in earlier work not included. Scalar features later re-emerged in work by Ladefoged (1971; see also discussion in Durand, 1990) among others, and unary features are found in several recent theoretical approaches, which are returned to later.

Another area of debate concerns equipollent and privative oppositions in feature theory (see further Durand 1990, p. 72; Harris, 1994, p. 92). An equipollent opposition is one where—with a binary feature—both the plus and minus values of the feature specify a particular property: That is to say the minus value does not imply mere absence of the feature but a different specification of it. For example, as noted by Durand (1990), the [+voice] feature refers to a particular glottal configuration; [−voice] should not be read as simply the lack of that glottal configuration, but needs to be understood as referring to a different glottal configuration: that needed to produce voicelessness.

On the other hand, a feature such as that proposed in Chomsky and Halle's (1968) *Sound Pattern of English* (SPE) for tongue height—[± high] —is arguably not equipollent, but privative. A privative opposition is one where the minus value of the feature is interpreted as mere absence of the plus, rather than as some configuration in its own right. If we consider vowel systems, the SPE feature [+high] is to be understood as referring to an oral configuration where the tongue is raised above a mid point and groups together as a natural class vowels such as /i, ü, u/. [−high], on the other hand, is not to be understood as a specific tongue position (e.g. lowered below a mid point), but rather as simply not raised above that mid point. The minus value of this feature, therefore,

---

[1]By this is meant phonologically. I return later to consider the difference between phonological and phonetic features.

can group both mid and low vowels together. The [±low] feature works in the same way, and by using these two we are able to isolate three different vowel heights: high [+high, –low], mid [–high, –low], and low [–high, +low]. The combination [+high, +low] is ruled out as being physically impossible.

That last point is worth considering further. Clearly, features whose very names appear to demonstrate how unlike they are, are not expected to be able to operate together to define a class of sounds. But the fact that the minus values can so operate demonstrates that the opposition for both these features is privative, not equipollent. An equipollent opposition might have allowed [–high] to represent, for example, a mid vowel tongue configuration, but not a low vowel one as well. As Harris (1994) points out, the position adopted in SPE was that features were uniformly expressed in terms of equipollent oppositions. Nevertheless, as our example has shown this was not always realized in fact, but as Durand (1990, p. 77) notes, "the possible defect of two interpretations of binary distinctive features . . . was discarded in the interests of formal unity."

Relationships Between Features

Another problem area concerns the relationships between features. For example, the feature [+sonorant] is much more likely to co-occur with the feature [+voice] than with [–voice]; the feature [+strident] has to co-occur with the feature [–sonorant]; the feature [+del rel] has to co-occur with [+consonantal] and so on. Classical SPE-type generative phonology attempted to deal with these relationships through markedness theory (again adapted from Prague School ideas). We do not have the space to go into this in any detail (see for example Durand's 1990 and Harris' 1994 discussions), but basically, markedness is an attempt to show which feature values and which feature combinations are more "natural" than others.[2] Natural, of course, may be interpreted as being a universal characteristic: Of phonologies of all languages; or it may be natural in terms of a given language. Markedness conventions, moreover, are external to the basic notation of generative phonology: They operate as a kind of mathematical table that is referred to in order to convert from u, and m values (unmarked and marked) to + and – ones. As Harris (1994, p. 93) points out, "a more radical solution is to build markedness relations directly into phonological representations," and goes on

[2]Underspecification theory can be thought of as having developed out of markedness approaches, but we do not have the space to follow those developments here (see Chapter 4, Roca, 1994, and van der Hulst and van de Weijer, 1995 for a fuller account of the development of underspecification).

to suggest that this is best done via a framework where phonological oppositions are uniformly privative.

Before turning to this point in more detail, we want to take a brief look at feature geometry (e.g., Clements, 1985; Sagey, 1986). In SPE, features were viewed as independent, but in more recent phonological work it has been recognized that dependency relations exist between features, as we have just noted. If features (whether of the SPE binary type or other privative types) are given some kind of dependency structure in terms of each other, then it will become easier to specify more from less natural phonological process. Roca (1994, p. 98), for example, notes that if all place features are gathered together into one node, then assimilation process such as found in many language between nasals and following obstruents can be expressed extremely simply and in such a way as to rule out only partial assimilation of place.

Those working within this area have constructed feature trees to express dependency relations between the wide range of features in SPE and post-SPE phonology (for some of the adaptations to features since SPE, see Roca, 1994). Feature geometry has proved a valuable tool in constraining the generative power of SPE type rules, but there is, of course, no reason why such formalism should be restricted to binary features of the type traditionally found in generative phonology.[3] Indeed, many recent studies have included some unary features in their trees (e.g., Sagey, 1986; Levelt, 1994), for example for place nodes such as labial, coronal, and dorsal. Indeed, Brown (1995) argues that considerations of theoretical parsimony would suggest that if some features are unary, then all should be. However, that does not mean that such unary features have direct phonetic interpretability, which is the claim of most of those referred to later.

Unary Components

In some comparatively recent work in phonology, the emphasis has shifted away from the use of equipollent, binary features to privative unary components. This can be seen within work in DP (see later and Anderson & Durand, 1986, 1987; Anderson & Ewen, 1987; Durand, 1990;

[3]We have not discussed at all developments in non-linear, or "tiered" phonology, as they do not bear directly on the debate as to what constitutes minimal units of phonology. Although autosegmental phonology does extract some aspects of description from a segmental tier and positions them on a higher tier, much of this structure can still be thought of in terms of traditional feature labels, or indeed—if desired—in terms of unary components. A review of the development of non-linear phonology is given in van der Hulst and van de Weijer (1995); see also Dinnsen, Chapter 4.

Lass, 1984), but also in other frameworks derived from DP (see, in particular, Harris, 1994; van der Hulst, 1989; Schane, 1995; Ewen, 1995 for references to other work). As noted, privative phonological components or elements[4] are ones which are either present—in which case the value of the unit is realized—or absent—in which case no alternative value is realized. There is, therefore, only one possible value associated with the unit, which is therefore shown to be unary as opposed to the binary possibilities of equipollent features.

Van der Hulst (1989) comments that the central motivation for a unary approach is that it constrains the phonology. Binary distinctive feature approaches allow a large number of natural classes (both + and – a feature), phonological systems, and processes. On the other hand, a unary system only allows, for example, classes of segments that share a component, not classes that do not share a component. As we saw earlier, markedness theory was an attempt within classical SPE phonology to constrain the over-richness of binary features. Harris (1994), too, sees unary accounts as ways of reducing the range of processes available to the theory to those that are observed in natural language data and thus avoiding theoretical add-ons (such as markedness conventions).[5]

There is a further claim made about unary components by many who work with them: that they have in fact phonetic interpretability, or at least that some of the components do (see van der Hulst, 1989, p. 261; Harris, 1994, p. 94). In any theory of phonological units below the level of the segment we may validly ask whether the units have independent phonetic

---

[4]In Dependency Phonology, these units are normally termed "components," whereas in Government Phonology the term "elements" is employed (see van der Hulst, 1989). The term "particle" is also encountered in Schane's work (e.g., Schane, 1995).

[5]Roca (1994) criticizes unary component accounts at least partly because of this constraining effect. He claims that certain naturally occurring processes cannot be accounted for just because there is no access to a negative aspect of a component. He cites the case of front and back high vowels that are involved in palatalization processes in certain languages; in DP terminology there is no prime that accounts for all high vowels: |i| and |u| are both needed. If a negative value of the prime |a| could be accessed, then a class of high vowels could be described via a single component. Clearly, this objection is only aimed at the arrangement of primes chosen in this particular framework (though, admittedly, it is commonly encountered in many approaches using unary components), rather than damning the unary approach as a whole. Further, various ways around this particular problem have been posited (see Anderson & Ewen, 1987; Ewen & van der Hulst, 1988). It must also be open to question whether every single phonological process must be seen to act on a single component; particularly when palatalization processes more often appear to act only with high front vowels. Harris (1994, p. 94) also comments that there is doubtless a corpus of robust equipollent accounts that need to be reassessed on a case-by-case basis in terms of an alternative privative account.

interpretation. In the case of traditional binary distinctive features, the answer is clearly negative. They may have phonetic content of some kind (for example, [+voice] as we noted earlier can be linked to an articulatory configuration), but this content can only manifest itself when joined with other feature values to fill the feature matrix of a specific segment. This means that these binary phonological features have at a late stage in the derivation to be mapped onto phonetic features (often viewed as multi-valued) for the string concerned to be interpreted phonetically.

Harris notes that a system of unary components where the components are phonetically interpretable primes means that at all levels of phonological derivation segments are phonetically interpretable (clearly not possible with underspecification approaches adopted in other theoretical stances; see Harris, 1994, pp. 94–95 for a detailed psycholinguistic critique of underspecification). That this is desirable becomes clear when we consider the roles of the phonology and phonetics in such an approach:

> Since phonological representation uniformly adheres to the principle of full phonetic interpretability, there is no motivation for recognizing an autonomous level of systematic phonetic representation. Any phonological representation at any level of derivation can be directly submitted to articulatory or perceptual interpretation. Derivation is thus not an operation by means of which abstract phonological objects are transformed into increasingly concrete physical objects. Rather it is a strictly generative function which defines the grammaticality of phonological strings. (Harris, 1994, p. 96)

Such a view of phonology differs from that held in traditional SPE-like accounts. As Harris claims, this structure, together with phonetically interpretable phonological elements may well be psycholinguistically more plausible. Recent developments in cognitive phonology (see Goldsmith, 1993; Bybee, 1994) have stressed psycholinguistic validity as a metric for phonological models. Interestingly, the contributors to the Goldsmith collection were more concerned with constraining the derivational process within a phonology (to fewer levels to mirror more closely what might be cognitively possible in terms of speech timing), and do not address the issue of what might be a cognitively valid smallest unit of phonological structure. Nevertheless, what we are tentatively claiming here is that unary privative components of the type described in this section are psycholinguistically more plausible than binary distinctive features.

DEPENDENCY PHONOLOGY

For the purposes of this chapter I intend to provide only a brief introduction to DP, concentrating on those aspects necessary for the analyses
to be presented later. As its name suggests, DP as a theory of phonology
is concerned with describing the relationships that hold between syllables, segments, segment features, and so on—in particular the relative
strengths or importance of these factors. Binary or multivalued features
are absent from DP; instead we have a set of unary components (see previous discussion), closely linked to the phonetics of speech production.
These components may be individually present, absent, or in combinations of various dependency types (see Anderson & Durand, 1986, p.
245; Anderson & Ewen, 1987, p. 151; Anderson & Durand, 1987).

Components are grouped into gestures, but there is as yet no complete agreement as to how these gestures are organized (Anderson &
Durand, 1986, p. 21). One account divides them into three groupings:
categorial, articulatory, and initiatory. Categorial covers consonantality,
voice, continuancy, and sonorance in traditional parlance; articulatory
covers place, height, rounding, backness, and nasality; and initiatory
covers glottal stricture, glottalicness, and velar suction.

Categorial Gesture

For the Categorial Gesture two components are suggested: " | V | , a com-
ponent which can be defined as 'relatively periodic', and | C | , a com-
ponent of 'periodic energy reduction'" (Anderson & Durand, 1986, p.
34). Combining these via various dependency relations gives us an
inventory of category types:

(1)   V   V   V   V,C   V:C   V:C   C   C
         | | | | |
         C   V,C   C   V   V
      vowels nasals liquids vls liq vcd frc vls frc vcd pls vls pls[6]

These configurations can also be shown in a simpler notation (from
Anderson & Durand, 1986; a slightly different version is employed in
Lass, 1984 and Anderson & Ewen, 1987):

(2)   { | V | }, { | V;C | }, { | V;V,C | }, { | V,C;C | }, { | V:C;V | }, { | V:C | }, { | C;V | }, { | C | }

---

[6]Affricates are deemed to be complex sounds and are returned to later in the chapter.

These notations are explained by Anderson and Durand (1986, p. 24):

> a notation employing unary components which may individually be absent, present, in simple combinations, or, if in combinations, either of equal or unequal strength.

And further

> Unary components may either be absent or present. If two components— a and b—are part of a gesture . . . they may enter into a simple combination (symbolized by a comma) . . . But they may enter into contrastive dependency relations whereby a governs b . . ., or b governs a . . ., or a and b mutually govern each other . . . government in the case of components is often symbolized in the DP literature by semi-colon for unilateral government . . . and by colon for mutual government.

Looking at (1) and (2), we can see that vowels are characterized by the component |V| ("relatively periodic") alone, whereas liquids are characterized by the component |V| governing the simple combination of |V| and |C| ("periodic energy reduction"). In other words, liquids are governed by sonorancy, with continuancy represented by the combination of |V| and |C|. (Other accounts suggest that {|V;V:C|} is a better motivated characterization of liquids, see Anderson and Ewen, 1987, but this difference need not detain us here.)

These sound types are deemed to be simple in that, although they contain further information (e.g. from the articulatory gesture), they lack any internal adjunction. DP describes various types of sounds that do show internal adjunction, and we can illustrate this process with a brief look at affricates and at diphthongs, although other sounds such as prenasalized stops can also be accounted for in a similar way.

Affricates, under this proposal, are deemed to have a stop notation to which is adjoined a fricative notation (rightwards to represent the fact that this friction occurs at the stop release)—as in (3), where information on the place of articulation would be shown in the empty brackets, the characteristics of voicing have been left unspecified:

(3) {|C;|}

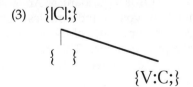

{ }

{V:C;}

Similar diagrams can be utilized to notate short diphthongs. Long diphthongs, as also long vowels, are considered to fill two slots in syllable structure (see following), but vowel systems lacking overt phonological vowel length distinctions (Anderson & Ewen, 1987 cite Scots English as a contemporary example) may still have diphthongal glides that need to be accounted for. These can be given the following notation:

(4) {|V|}

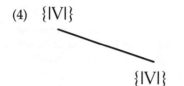

{|V|}

Initiatory Gesture

Although the categories in (1) and (2) above represent many of the speech sounds likely to be encountered in disordered speech data, there are some types not included. One such is the voiceless nasal type, that can be found in cleft palate speech, as well as in children's speech where voiceless nasals often occur as reflexes of /s/+nasal initial clusters (frequently termed "feature synthesis" or "coalescence"). To cope with these DP utilizes the Initiatory Gesture, and in particular the component |O| ("glottal opening") (see Ewen, 1982a, b, p. 88; Lass, 1984, p. 290; Anderson & Durand, 1986, p. 40). Other components of this gesture exist to cope with nonpulmonic sounds, and we return to these later. We will follow the usage of this component set out in Anderson and Durand (1986) who show the use of the Initiatory Gesture along with the Categorial Gesture in, for example, vowels:

(5) V
 |
 O
 vowels

Normally, however, the inclusion of |O| is redundant: as Anderson and Ewen (1987, p. 192) state, "while both voiced and voiceless sonorants will display |O| phonetically, . . . one member of the opposition lacks the component in phonological representations." This member for sonorants is the voiced one, capturing the difference in naturalness between voiced and voiceless sonorants.

Obstruents can, of course, occur as both voiced and voiceless: but here the distinction is well captured via the |V| and |C| components, so here too | O | is usually redundant (although it can, of course, be utilized for full phonetic specifications). It is needed, however, to show aspirated stops and /h/ ({| O;C|} and {| O;V|} respectively; see Lass, 1984, p. 289; Anderson and Ewen, 1987, p. 193).

We noted above that voiceless nasals needed the | O | component to be marked in their representation. For these sounds, Anderson and Durand suggest (1986, p. 40):

(6)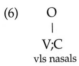

where the "glottal opening" component governs | V |, which in turn governs | C |. Compared with voiced nasals, we see the addition of the | O | component into the phonological representation. How might this explain the commonly found feature synthesis previously referred to? If we show the full Initiatory Gesture description for voiceless fricatives (see Ewen, 1982a for other circumstances when such a full description is useful), we will see how the feature synthesis process noted does indeed see the combination of the | O |-ness of the fricative with the Categorial dependency relations of the nasal (we ignore in this example nonlinear aspects of the characterization of this cluster):

(7)
$$
\begin{array}{ccccc}
\text{O} & & \text{V,O} & & \text{O} \\
| & + & | & \rightarrow & | \\
\text{V:C} & & \text{V;C} & & \text{V;C} \\
\text{vls fric} & & \text{vcd nasal} & & \text{vls nasal}
\end{array}
$$

We can use this gesture, too, to account for different phonation types apart from the voiced-voiceless distinction. In some languages, phonation types such as breathy and creaky are used contrastively, so need to be captured in any phonological description. They may also be used noncontrastively or as part of a voice disorder, where the phonetic level of description will still need to account for them. As Anderson and Ewen (1987) point out, languages use a maximum of three different phonation types contrastively, therefore the | O | component can be utilized to distinguish these three in a relative manner: That is to say particular combinations of components can represent different phonation types dependant on the set of types to be distinguished. If a distinction is needed between voiceless, breathy and voiced phonation, the following notation is posited:

(8)   {O}   {O}:{|C|;}   {|C|;}
         | |
      {|C|;}   {O}
     voiceless   breathy   voiced

If, on the other hand, the contrast was between voiceless, voiced and creaky, the notation would signify different phonation types:

(9)   {O}   {O}:{|C|;}   {|C|;}
         | |
      {|C|;}   {O}
     voiceless   voiced   creak

This gesture is also concerned with the characterization of nonpulmonic airstream mechanisms. Anderson and Ewen (1987) note that the presence of |O| in the phonological or phonetic description of a segment automatically implies the use of a pulmonic airstream. However, three other airstreams can be encountered in natural language: glottalic egressive and ingressive, and velaric ingressive (giving us ejectives, implosives, and clicks in traditional phonetic parlance). A component of "glottalicness" (symbolized by |G|) is set up to account for ejectives and implosives. As with the |O| component, |G| can enter into dependency relations with the categorial gesture, and it is proposed, therefore, that ejectives are characterized by |G| governing an item of the categorial gesture. For ejective stops, fricatives, and affricates this would be as in (10):

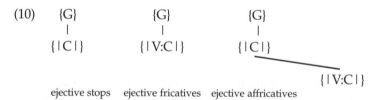

(10)   {G}   {G}   {G}
         | | |
       {|C|}   {|V:C|}   {|C|}
                                                       {|V:C|}
     ejective stops   ejective fricatives   ejective affricatives

Implosives, on the other hand, involve an ingressive airstream, and to account for this, DP formalism reverses the governing relationship between the |G| component and the categorial gesture. Implosives (as the name suggests) occur only with oral stop type consonants in natural language, thus, a voiceless implosive would be described as in:

(11)   {|C|}
         |
        {G}

However, we mostly encounter implosives using a mixture of glottalic ingressive air and pulmonic egressive air (see Ball, 1993), which gives us voiced implosives. These are characterized by a combination of the |G| and |O| components:

(12) {O,G}
   |
   {|C|;}
   voiced implosive

In this last example, as both |O| and |G| can only be present in voiced implosives, the direction of the governing relationship between these components of the initiatory gesture, and the component of the categorial gesture are not important. Indeed, going back to our examples of breathy voice and creaky voice types in (8) and (9) above, we can see how breathy and creaky versions of implosives could be characterized:

(13) {O,G}   {|C;|}
   | |
   {|C|;}   {O,G}
   breathy voiced   creaky voiced implosives

The velaric ingressive airstream mechanism produces the so-called click sounds. DP uses the component |K| to characterize the use of this mechanism. In languages that employ clicks, simultaneous pulmonic egressive activity may also be used to create sound types termed "nasalized clicks", "aspirated clicks" and so on. Some of these types, together with the normal click (deemed to involve lack of aspiration) are shown in (14) (aspirated click, delayed aspirated click, unaspirated click, click with glottal stop):

(14) {O,K}   {O,K}:{|C|}   {|C|}   {K},{|C|}
   | |
   {|C|}   {O,K}
   /ǃ͡h/   /ǃh/   /ǃ/   /ǃʔ/[7]

---

[7]The transcriptions in Anderson and Ewen (1987) employ the formalism of Ladefoged and Traill (1984), whereby clicks are usually shown as co-occurring with /k/. This means that the transcriptions for the four types in example (14) are given by these authors as: /kǃh/ /ǃh/ /kǃ/ /ǃʔ/.

Articulatory Gesture

The third level of representation is the Articulatory Gesture. This gesture deals with place of articulation for vowels and for consonants and aspects such as orality-nasality, central versus lateral release, and secondary and double articulations. In this chapter, the most important of the components for this gesture are noted briefly.

For vowels, are found the components:

|i| frontness

|a| lowness

|u| roundness

|ə| centrality

The treatment of back unrounded vowels is not completely settled, but according to Anderson and Ewen (1987) does not require other components as has been proposed, but can be accounted for with the above components. Examples of representations of different vowels and the dependency relations of the components can be seen as:

(15) |i| |i;a| |i:a| |a;i|
       [i]   [e]   [ɛ]   [a]

       |u| |u;a| |u:a| |a;u|
       [u]   [o]   [ɔ]   [ɒ]

       |i,u| |ə| |a| |ə:i,u|
       [y]   [ɨ]   [ɐ]   [ɯ]

For consonants, the following main components are found:

|u| roundness/gravity

|l| linguality

|t| apicality

|d| dentality

|r| retracted tongue root

|α| advanced tongue root

|λ| laterality

|n| nasality

To show how the place components combine in different dependency relations to represent place of articulation, we can examine a range of nasal consonants:

(16) | u,n | | u,d,n | | l,d,n | | l;t,n | | t;l,n |
      [m]   [m̩]   [n̪]   [n]   [n̺]

      | l,i,n | | l,u,n | | l,u,a,n |
      [ɲ]   [ŋ]   [ɴ]

In this brief review of DP, we have concentrated on the representation of segments, and have ignored the structures proposed for syllables, and for accounting for stress and tone and so on, due to pressures of space. In the following section we examine some examples of commonly occurring phonological changes in disordered speech, and attempt to show the advantages of a DP account over more traditional accounts.

DP AND DISORDERED SPEECH

We saw earlier how DP could account elegantly for the feature synthesis process sometime encountered in child speech and in disordered speech. In the rest of the chapter, I hope to demonstrate how DP can account for some other commonly found aspects of disordered phonology. We have space only to examine the following three: fricative stopping, velar fronting, and liquid gliding.

Fricative stopping involves the realization of target fricatives as plosives at the nearest place of articulation. There is therefore a class change but no change in place or voicing. If we return to the representations of different sound types given in (1) and (2), we can initially draw up a description of the changes here in DP terms as follows:

(17) **a.** { | V:C;V | }   →   { | C;V | }
           voiced fricatives   →   voiced plosives

      b. { | V:C | }   →   { | C | }
           voiceless fricatives   →   voiceless plosives

Clearly, this will be more economical if we can combine both (17a) and (17b) into a single description, and DP formalism allows us to do this by combining those components that are held in common by the sound groups in question. Adopting this procedure we can rephrase (17) as (18):

(18)   {|V:C;|}   →   {|C|;}

This description clearly shows that the change involved here is the loss of the mutually governing |V| component to leave |C| alone (irrespective of what might be governed by that |C|). The representation of plosive by {|C|;} is a means of showing that |C| alone is found in governing position, and that this is the necessary condition to distinguish the plosive group from obstruents as a whole.

It might be argued that (18) is simply another way of representing a more traditional SPE type of rule:

(19)   [+continuant]   →   [–continuant] / $\begin{bmatrix} +\text{consonantal} \\ -\text{vocalic} \end{bmatrix}$

However, although rule (19) notes the change from the positive to the negative value for a binary feature (i.e., that a particular aspect is present or absent), the DP approach is more versatile, in that it shows the change in the relationship between components: that a mutual government of |V| and |C| changes to the |C| alone: i.e., an increase in the influence of a particular component as opposed to the mere presence versus absence of a feature. How does this approach help in clinical phonology?

This particular instance requires therapy to concentrate on production of articulatory strictures that avoid a complete blockage to oral airflow, in other words the production of a narrow channel to cause turbulent airflow. At the phonological level for this instance it is probably not very important whether this task is characterized as one of plus or minus a feature, or one of a change in dependency relations between components. However, a process like fricative stopping is in reality one part of a hierarchy of fortition whereby classes of sounds become "stronger" or more "fortis." This process, and indeed the opposite one of lenition, is encountered frequently in clinical phonology, and as noted in Lass (1984) DP is particularly suited to characterizing these changes, as each step shows one more change in dependency relations between maximum |V| at one end and maximum |C| at the other. In therapeutic terms, this serves to make explicit for clinicians the need to view classes of sounds as part of a continuum where particular phonetic aspects (such as voice and manner of articulation) are on a cline rather than being a matter of simple presence versus absence. (20) illustrates a fortition-lenition hierarchy in DP terms:

(20) a.

```
                          O                          O
                          |                          |
         o   C    ↔    C    ↔   V:C    ↔    V
         p   ↕         ↕         ↕          ↕
         e
         n   C    ↔   V,C    ↔    V     ↔    V
         i   |          |         |
         n
         g   V          V        V:C
                   sonorization
```

b.

```
              k    ↔    kʰ    ↔    x     ↔    h
              ↕         ↕         ↕          ↕
              g    ↔    ɣ    ↔    w     ↔    u
```

Although the fricative to plosive change reported earlier can be accounted for as part of a fortition process, that is the dependency relations among components shows an increase in the power of $|C|$, we can also find lenition processes, for example in dysarthric speech where weakening of stops to fricatives or to approximants is common. In this case, we see an increase in the power of $|V|$. Ewen (1982b), Ball (1990), and Ball and Müller (1993) take a DP approach to lenition in natural language.

A second commonly occurring phonological change in disordered speech data is often termed velar fronting. In this process we find velar plosives and the velar nasal realized (most commonly) as alveolars. In languages where velar fricatives occur, these may also be affected, but evidence is somewhat scarce here. In accounting for this change, DP would only utilize components from the Articulatory Gesture, as manner of articulation and voice is preserved (assuming, of course, that interaction from other changes is not also present). We can show the change involved in velar fronting as:

(21) $\{|l,u|\}$ → $\{|l;t|\}$

This representation demonstrates that two changes have in fact taken place. First, we see that the gravity component that is present with the lingual component in velars in a nongoverning relationship has been dropped, and, secondly, that a different component (apicality) is brought into alveolars, dependent on linguality. In other words, not only have we exchanged two components in this process, but we have changed the dependency relationships between linguality and the other component.

To explore how this differs from a binary feature approach we can look at velar fronting as expressed in a generative phonological format:

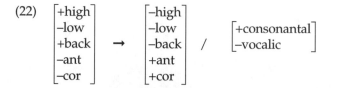

(22)
$$
\begin{bmatrix} +\text{high} \\ -\text{low} \\ +\text{back} \\ -\text{ant} \\ -\text{cor} \end{bmatrix} \rightarrow \begin{bmatrix} -\text{high} \\ -\text{low} \\ -\text{back} \\ +\text{ant} \\ +\text{cor} \end{bmatrix} \bigg/ \begin{bmatrix} +\text{consonantal} \\ -\text{vocalic} \end{bmatrix}
$$

This rule involves changing the feature values of four of the five place features to express the move from velar to alveolar, and is therefore considerably less simple than the DP approach. Further, for the therapist planning a remediation program, the DP analysis overtly specifies the target for intervention—that is working on eliminating apicality for the target velars and replacing that with lingual gravity—in other words raising of the back of the tongue. The rule in (22), if taken as an input to a scheme of remediation would suggest the need to work on four different aspects of articulation to achieve the desired place.

The third aspect we will examine is that traditionally termed "liquid gliding" (see Grunwell, 1986). The most commonly encountered manifestation of this is the change from target /r/ (=[ɹ]) to [w] (or sometimes [ʋ]), found in normal phonological development as well as in phonological disorders. In terms of distinctive features, this change involves not only a change of major class (from liquid to glide), but also a change in place of articulation. Grunwell (1986) points out that a full specification of this change involves altering the values of five features, with a further one feature each required for the individual sounds. We can show this in (23) below, where the asterisks mark the feature differences between the target and the realization:

(23)
$$
\begin{bmatrix} +\text{son} \\ +\text{syll} \\ +\text{cons} \\ -\text{ant} \\ +\text{cor} \\ -\text{high} \\ -\text{low} \\ -\text{back} \\ -\text{nasal} \\ +\text{cont} \\ -\text{strid} \\ +\text{voice} \\ -\text{lat} \\ \underline{\quad\quad} \end{bmatrix} \rightarrow \begin{bmatrix} +\text{son} \\ -\text{syll*} \\ -\text{cons*} \\ -\text{ant} \\ -\text{cor*} \\ +\text{high*} \\ -\text{low} \\ +\text{back*} \\ -\text{nasal} \\ +\text{cont} \\ -\text{strid} \\ +\text{voice} \\ \underline{\quad\quad}\text{*} \\ +\text{round*} \end{bmatrix}
$$

The fact that such a commonly occurring sound change requires such a complex set of feature changes is counterintuitive, as Grunwell (1986) notes. We will now look at how a DP approach differs from the change in (23). First, DP does not recognize the distinction between glides and liquids of traditional distinctive feature approaches. These two sound types are both subsumed within the liquid category, equivalent in phonetic parlance to the approximant type. This means that no change is needed in the components of the Categorial Gesture, only in the Articulatory Gesture. The components required to specify the usual approximant /r/ of most English accents will depend upon whether the articulation is considered most similar to alveolar or to retroflex. As there is often a degree of retroflexion to the tongue tip, we will assume the latter. This gives us a change as shown in (24):

(24) {|t:l|} → {|l,u|,|u|}

This change is more complex than those shown in previous examples, but is nevertheless considerably simpler than that shown in (23). Here we see the addition of an extra roundness component showing that [w] is a doubly articulated sound, and the change of linguality from being governed by apicality (to give retroflexion) to existing together with gravity to show velar position. For ease of explication, we have omitted from (24) the Categorial Gesture components that mark liquids.

This account again directly informs the therapist's remediation in a way that (23) cannot. It shows overtly and explicitly the change from a simple approximant to a doubly articulated one, and the change in tongue position. This means that therapy must involve the replacement of the gravity found with the velar approximation, and the institution of a retroflex approximation. The fact that /r/ in many English accents has a secondary rounding can make an even clearer comparison of the two sounds. Secondary characteristics are shown governed by the primary, so we can see an alternative version of (24) in (24'):

(24') {|t:l|} → {|l,u|,|u|}
          |
          u

This characterization suggests that the change has involved a raising in status of the |u| component, such that not only is it instituted as an independent component, but that it also affects the lingual component. It can even be argued that (24') gives a phonological motivation for the change in that a representation of government is replaced by a less complex representation of simple combination.

DEPENDENCY PHONOLOGY
ABOVE THE SEGMENT

However, DP is not solely concerned with representation at the segmental level, but like many recent developments in phonological theory, it presents analysis at higher levels, such as the syllable, foot, word, and utterance. We do not have the time here to go into all these in great detail, but will consider a couple of examples which have particular relevance to disordered speech.

As with components at the segmental level, differing dependency relations can hold between elements on higher levels (though at these levels it is simply a choice between governing and nongoverning, as in GP described later); in DP formalism these are usually expressed through linear diagrams of the sort made familiar by various non-linear approaches to phonology (see Dinnsen, this volume). Some of the conditions described in the DP literature (e.g., Anderson, 1986) on suprasegmental structure are quite complex and need not detain us here. We can, firstly, illustrate a few typical syllable structure patterns, which can lead in to a brief discussion of disordered speech at this level.

Diagrams (25), (26), and (27) represent syllable graphs for three different types of initial consonant clusters in English. These representations are assigned the following conventions, or rules, on rhyme and syllable formation (e.g. Anderson and Ewen, 1987, pp. 108–109) given in (28) and (29), and account for the differences in sonority values between /s/+stop clusters and stop+liquid clusters (i.e., differences in dependency relations between the segments).

(25)

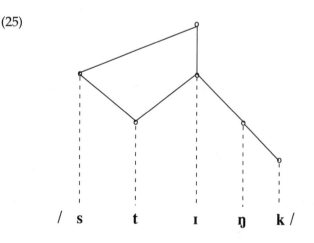

/ s   t   ɪ   ŋ   k /

(26)

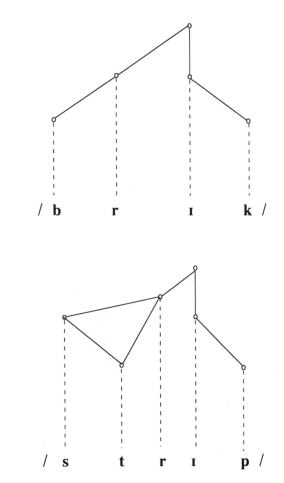

/ b   r   ɪ   k /

(27)

/ s   t   r   ɪ   p /

A cluster reduction strategy, common in language acquisition and phonological delay and disorder, can be accounted for by alterations to the syllable rules (see 28′ and 29′ and figures in 25′, 26′, and 27′). We can envisage alterations to the rules restricting their application to certain segment types and thus decoupling certain of the consonants in the target cluster. It might also be considered that simplification of the more complex /s/+stop clusters (in sonority and dependency terms) could be expressed in terms of alterations to both the rhyme and the syllable formation conventions to rule out two direct governing relations, or, perhaps, rule out a segment being both a governor and being governed (as is /s/ in these cases), or as shown in (28′) and (29′), by appealing to the

(25')

(26')

(27')

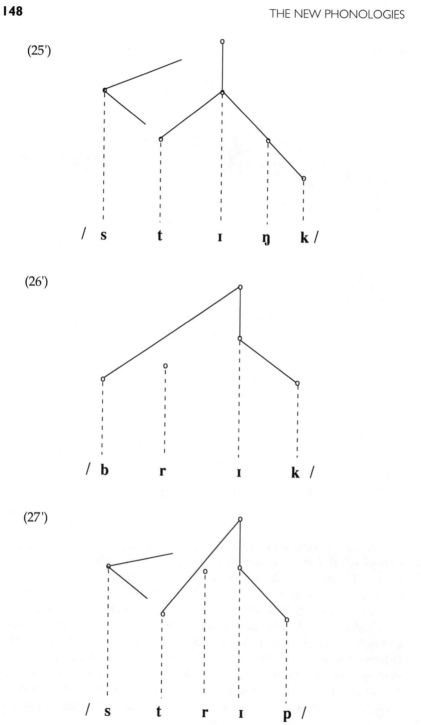

category (i.e. consonant) of governing and governed items. Stop+liquid clusters are often reported as being acquired first in both normal language acquisition and in child language intervention, and we can see that with these clusters the simple extension of the syllable formation rule is required, while for /s/+stop clusters full versions of both rules are required to interact.

We can also see, in (30), how the alteration of these conventions—in this instance through the removal of the rhyme-formation rule—can result in the decoupling of the coda to a syllable, with final consonant deletion as another commonly occurring process.

We can consider also the problem of other /s/+ initial cluster types in English in both phonological acquisition and disordered phonology. The most common of these are /sm-/, /sn-/, /sl-/ and /sw-/. If we look at the sonority hierarchy of sound categories as shown in (1) and (2), it is easy to see that both nasals and liquids[8] are higher in sonority than voiceless fricatives. This means that syllable graphs for these clusters are going to resemble the stop+liquid type rather than the /s/+stop type. We can illustrate this in (31), with a syllable representation of the word "snap."

We would expect, therefore, that cluster reduction strategies with these clusters would take the form of the amended version of syllable formation ((29')), that is a decoupling of the liquid. Indeed, Grunwell (1986) does note that forms such as [sæp] for /snæp/ do occur. However, it appears that forms such as [næp] may also be found.[9] The difference in sonority values between the items in the target cluster is clearly not as great as between stops and liquids; it may be, therefore, that for some children and disordered speakers the strategy employed with /s/+stop clusters is extended through analogy to other /s/+ clusters, although for others the strategy employed with stop+liquid clusters is extended to /s/+liquid/nasal clusters.

Syllable Formation Rules

(Anderson & Ewen, 1987, pp. 108–109)

(28) Rhyme formation
      Given segments a, b, where a<<b, a $\rightleftarrows$ b if b is weak, i.e. is not more sonorous than a.

---

[8]As noted, in DP, both traditionally termed liquids and glides (phonetically, the approximants) are termed liquids.

[9]We noted earlier that coalescence of target cluster items into a single new segment may also occur (see (7)). This discussion is only concerned with cluster reduction possibilities.

(29)   Syllable formation
Given segments a, b, where a≤b, a ⇸ b by (28), b ⇉ a.

(28′)   Rhyme formation (amended)
Given segments a, b, where a<<b, , a ⇉ b if b is weak, i.e., is
not more sonorous than a. *if a = {C} and if ⇸ a, decouple a.*

(29′)   Syllable formation (amended)
Given segments a, b, where a≤≤b, and a ⇉ b by (28),
b ⇉ a. *if b = {C}, decouple a.*

(30)

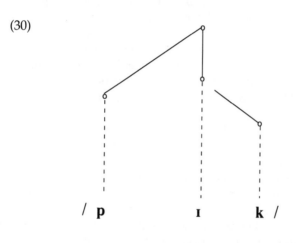

/ **p**   ɪ   **k** /

(31)

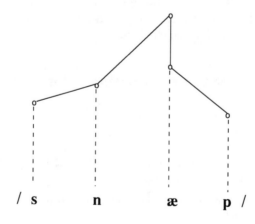

/ **s**   **n**   **æ**   **p** /

Weak syllable deletion, processes affecting stress placement, and intonation can all be accounted for in DP terms. Details of the treatment of stress and of word structure generally can be found in Anderson and Ewen (1987, p. 96); again, they take the form of tree structures illustrating dependency relations between aspects of word structure. A process like weak syllable deletion can also, therefore, be characterized in terms of the simplification of such a tree.

GOVERNMENT PHONOLOGY (GP)

Government Phonology (Kaye, Lowenstamm, & Vergnaud, 1985, 1990; Harris, 1990, 1994; Harris & Lindsey, 1995) can be viewed to some extent as an off-shoot of DP, prompted at least in part by a desire to constrain the over-generative power of the former approach. That DP allows four different dependency relations (non-governing, mutual governing, a governing b, and b governing a), and a relatively high number of phonological units, means that a large number of phonological relations can be generated by the theory. This can be seen as a disadvantage, as it is likely to produce more combinations than are needed to characterize natural language. (However, we must bear in mind that this may to some extent be useful in the description of atypical speech.) Successor theories to DP, therefore, were concerned to some extent to reduce both the number of relationships allowed to hold between units and the number of units themselves. This is still an area of controversy (see later), but we briefly outline a version of GP that has been featured in the recent literature.

John Harris in several recent publications (e.g. 1994; Harris & Lindsey, 1995) develops a version of Government Phonology where the atoms of phonological structure clearly owe a lot to DP as described earlier, but also to other developments in phonological theory—notably feature geometry (e.g., Clements, 1985; Sagey, 1986). One of Harris's initial concerns in his 1994 publication is to argue for unary phonological primes, as opposed to the traditional binary distinctive features of most approaches to phonology since Chomsky and Halle (1968). This, of course, is also a characteristic of the DP approach and has been discussed in some detail earlier.

As with DP, GP has concerns at the level of the word and above, and these are described clearly in Brockhaus (1995). There are also broader phonological concerns, such as the status of derivation and

interfaces between phonology and the lexicon and phonology and phonetics, and these are discussed in Harris and Lindsey (1995) and Kaye
(1995). We concentrate in this section, however, on the elements of
phonological structure (sometimes termed the "melodic primes"), as
this will give us the most direct comparison with those aspects of DP
that we concentrated on earlier in this chapter. Originally, Kaye et al.
(1985, 1990) proposed ten active elements used in defining segmental
expressions[10]:

A	non-high	**R**	coronal
U	labial/round	**?**	occluded
I	front/palatal	**h**	aperiodic energy (noise)
Ɨ	ATR	**H**	stiff vocal cords
N	nasal	**L**	slack vocal cords

Since Kaye et al.'s publications, there has been considerable debate
within the GP literature as to the desirability of reducing the number of
elements in order to constrain the generative power of the theory.
Reductions to seven, five, and (as we note later) two elements have all
been proposed (see Ritter, 1996; van der Hulst, 1993, 1994, 1995, 1996).
The ATR element is generally realized in alternative ways in current
models of the theory (see Harris & Lindsey, 1995), and it has also been
suggested that the nasal element can be dispensed with, with nasals
being described perhaps through using the L element heading (i.e., governing[11]) the relevant place element (in a similar way to the approach of
DP). The attempt to eliminate **R**, **?**, and **h** is also noted in Ritter (1996),
though this step is perhaps less convincing. Harris (1994) and Harris
and Lindsey (1995) both retain these elements, and point to the fact that
the acoustic record supports this retention, in that clear acoustic correlates of both the place features and the manner features are found. Harris and Lindsey (1995) note that elements, in a full account, would be
placed on separate autosegmental tiers, but we do not have space to
pursue this area further.

---

[10]It should be noted that in GP these elements are deemed to be phonetically interpretable
at all stages of derivation. This results in radical differences in the role of phonological
derivation and the loss of a level of systematic phonetics (see Harris & Lindsey, 1995).

[11]Early version of GP used the notion of "charm" to characterize which elements were
governors and which were governed (see Kaye, et al., 1985, 1990; Harris, 1990). This system is no longer found in much of the recent literature.

Following Harris (1994), therefore, we can present an "element geometry" tree of the elements found in that approach to GP in (32):

(32)

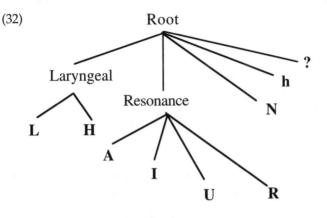

(In Harris & Lindsey, 1995, the **N** node is deleted.)

To see how these elements are used to describe particular segments, we can examine a selection of both vowels and consonants. Harris (1994) assumes a prime @ that represented centrality in vowels and dorsal (but non-palatal) in consonants, that is to represent velar.[12]

Vowels

Vowels represented by the simple three vowel elements are:

(33)   **A**   [a][13]
          I   [i]
          U   [u]

Combinations of elements will provide a wider vowel set, of course. However, in combinations, one element is normally deemed to be the "head" (or governor) and others are dependent on the head. In

[12]@ was omitted from the tree because it represents a default value or "blank canvas" (Harris, personal communication).

[13]The vowel here is presumed to be somewhere between cardinal vowel 4 and 5. In this and other lists of symbols, IPA values are followed. In Harris (1994) and Harris and Lindsey (1995) the Americanist tradition is adhered to.

GP formalism the head element is underlined; where no element is underlined, then the elements are in non-governing relationship. Unlike DP, GP does not utilize the mutual governing relationship. If we examine some English vowels, we can see this process in operation:

(34) **[I, @]**   /ɪ/
      [A, I, @]   /ɛ/
      [I, A]   /æ/
      [U, A]   /ɒ/
      [U, @]   /ʊ/
      [@]   /ʌ/
      [A, @]   [ɐ]

As can be seen, those short vowels of English that are generally considered to be lax vowels as well, are governed by the neutral element @. Looking at long vowels, it should be noted that in GP these are considered to occupy two segment slots (like diphthongs), and can be characterized as follows:[14]

(35)

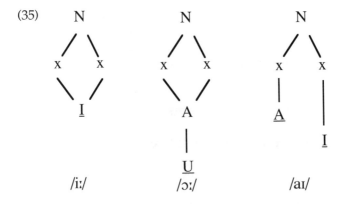

Turning now to consonants, we can give (as with vowels) the phonetic interpretation of the elements most frequently used to characterize them. It should be noted that the slightly different exponence of the **I** and the **U** elements derives from their no longer being dominated by a nucleus node in word structure.

[14]N in the following diagrams stands for nucleus, not the nasal element.

Consonants

?	?
h	h
R	ɾ
I	j
U	w
@	ɰ
A	ʁ̝

The following can serve as illustrations of the use of both place and manner features in a range of consonants (these examples are all voiceless to avoid the inclusion of the laryngeal node elements that control the voicing distinction among other aspects):

(36)   [h, U, ?]   p
        [h, R, ?]   t
        [h, @, ?]   k
        [h, U]   f
        [h, R]   s
        [h, R]   θ
        [h, R, I]   ʃ   (alternatively [h, I])
        [h, @]   x
        [h, A]   χ
        [h, A]   ħ
        [R, ?]   l

Other consonants found in English are included above as the exponence of the simple elements, although consonants such as nasals can be characterized through the inclusion of the element **N** (see Ritter, 1996 for an alternative to avoid the use of this element).

GP as a Description of Disordered Phonology

Unlike Dependency Phonology, Government Phonology has not yet been used to any extent in the description of disordered speech. However, it has been used to describe many historical phonological processes (see Harris, 1994), and phonological acquisition (see Ball, 1996; Harrison, 1996) so we could easily extend those kinds of analyses to processes in disordered speech.

First, vowel errors of those who have postlingual hearing impairment (see Ball, 1993) show patterns of mid vowel raising to close positions with both front and back vowels and for lower mid vowels there is a process of vowel lowering to open positions, again affecting front and back vowels. In a GP account of such processes, we see a simplification of the segmental description, with vowels becoming progressively more like **I**, **U**, or **A**.

(37) [A, I, @]   →   [I, @]   →   [I]
      /ɛ/   →   /ɪ/   →   /i/
      [A, U]   →   [A, U]   →   [A]
      /ɔ/   →   /ɒ/   →   /ɑ/

As shown during the discussion of DP, lenition and fortition processes of consonants are both found in disordered speech: fortition in such processes as fricative stopping and lenition in the weakening found in some dysarthric speech. In GP, as in DP, both fortition and lenition can be characterized as the progressive adding or deleting of elements or the alteration of dependency relations between elements. The lenition of /t/ is illustrated in (38) (the fortition would of course require the reversal of the steps shown), with x standing for the consonantal place in structure:

(38) t   →   s   →   h   →   Ø
      x   x   x   (x)
      | | |
      h   h   h
      | |
      R   R
      |
      ?

This process, then, is seen as the gradual elimination of melodic material until an empty slot is obtained. In terms of processes such as fricative stopping we are assuming that an element such as **?** is attached to all consonantal nodes, and the removal of such an element is accomplished at a later stage of phonological development (and in the case of disordered phonology, may not be accomplished). This differs from traditional SPE-type feature approaches, where it is assumed an extra feature such as [continuant] has to be learned, and has echoes, perhaps, of approaches such as Natural Phonology (see Grunwell, Chapter 3).

It will be interesting to see whether GP, with its expanding popularity in theoretical phonology, will be applied in detail to clinical phonology, and whether such an application will modify the theory in interesting ways.

RADICAL cv PHONOLOGY

Radical cv Phonology (see van der Hulst, 1993, 1994, 1995, 1996) is claimed by van der Hulst to be a development from Dependency Phonology, but one that relies solely on two elements (C and V), and four combinations of elements (C, V, C_V, V_C). It is a new and still developing approach to phonology, and so only a brief sketch of a small part of the theory is given. This will look at the characterization of the segment, so we can directly compare it to the accounts given earlier in this chapter.

Clearly, reducing the number of elements to two requires greater depth of analysis of constructs such as the segment. In Radical cv Phonology, therefore, the segment is considered to structure hierarchically into three main components (the specifier, the head, and the complement); in turn, the head and complement are divided into a further three components. At each of these levels, we find the C and V elements and their possible combinations. The two elements, therefore, provide us with a much larger number of possible phonological contrasts. The Segment Hierarchy (taken from van der Hulst, 1996) is shown in (39).[15]

We have not touched here on structures above the segment, nor on the applicability of such an approach to the characterization of disordered speech. This account, however, may well appeal to clinical phonologists and clinicians, due to its very simplicity at the element level, and one can only look forward to further work in this theory.

CONCLUSION

In this chapter we have attempted to describe and illustrate current thinking in phonological theories that adopt a monovalent approach to minimal phonological units. Although DP is the longest standing of the theories discussed, and has been applied to disordered as well as normal speech, it has recently come under pressure due to its generous generative power. We have seen the current quest for ever more constrained phonologies, and it is to be hoped that clinical phonologists, with their

---

[15]In (39) the abbreviations represent the following: SPEC: specifier; COMPL: complement; Phon: phonation; Strict: stricture; SecPla: secondary place; MajPla: major place; SubPla: subordinate place; hi-mi: high-mid; lo-mi: low-mid; constr.: constricted glottis; aspir.: aspirated; fric: fricative; approx: approximant; lat: lateral; stri/rho: strident/rhotic; voi/atr: voice/advanced tongue root; palat.: palatalized; labial.: labialized; dorsal.: dorsalized; pharyng.: pharyngealized; poster.: posterior.

(39)   The Segment

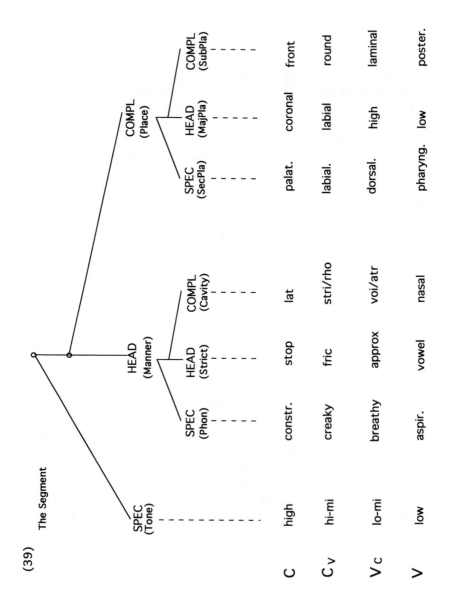

	SPEC (Tone)	SPEC (Phon)	HEAD (Strict)	COMPL (Cavity)	SPEC (SecPla)	HEAD (MajPla)	COMPL (SubPla)
C	high	constr.	stop	lat	palat.	coronal	front
C_V	hi-mi	creaky	fric	stri/rho	labial.	labial	round
V_C	lo-mi	breathy	approx	voi/atr	dorsal.	high	laminal
V	low	aspir.	vowel	nasal	pharyng.	low	poster.

fascinating data sets, will join in the debate as to how constrained a theory should be.

REFERENCES

Anderson, J. (1986). Suprasegmental dependencies. In J. Durand (Ed.), *Dependency and non-linear phonology* (pp. 55–133). London: Croom Helm.

Anderson, J., & Durand, J. (1986). Dependency phonology. In J. Durand, (Ed.), *Dependency and non-linear phonology* (pp. 1–54). London: Croom Helm.

Anderson, J., & Durand, J. (Eds.). (1987). *Explorations in dependency phonology.* Dordrecht: Foris.

Anderson, J., & Ewen, C. (1987). *Principles of dependency phonology.* Cambridge, England: Cambridge University Press.

Ball, M. J. (1990). The lateral fricative: Lateral or fricative. In M. J. Ball, J. Fife, E. Poppe, & J. Rowland (Eds.), *Celtic linguistics/ Ieithyddiaeth geltaidd: Readings in the Brythonic languages: Festschrift for T. Arwyn Watkins* (pp. 109–125). Amsterdam: John Benjamins.

Ball, M. J. (1993). *Phonetics for speech pathology* (2nd ed.). London: Whurr.

Ball, M. J. (1996). An examination of the nature of the minimal phonological unit in language acquisition. In B. Bernhardt, J. Gilbert, & D. Ingram (Eds.), *Proceedings of the UBC International Conference on Phonological Acquisition* (pp. 240–253). Somerville, MA: Cascadilla Press.

Ball, M. J., & Müller, N. (1993). *Mutation in Welsh.* London: Routledge.

Brockhaus, W. (1995). Skeletal and suprasegmental structure within government phonology. In J. Durand & F. Katamba (Eds.), *Frontiers of phonology* (pp. 180–221). London: Longmans.

Brown, C. (1995). The feature geometry of lateral approximants and lateral fricatives. In H. van der Hulst & J. van de Weijer (Eds.), *Leiden in last* (pp. 41–88). The Hague: Holland Academic Graphics.

Bybee, J. (1994). A view of phonology from a cognitive and functional perspective. *Cognitive Linguistics, 5,* 285–305.

Chomsky, N., & Halle, M. (1968). *The sound pattern of English.* Cambridge, MA: MIT Press.

Clements, G. (1985). The geometry of phonological features. *Phonology Yearbook, 2,* 225–252.

Durand, J. (1990). *Generative and non-linear phonology.* London: Longmans.

Ewen, C. (1982a). The internal structure of complex segments. In H. van der Hulst & N. Smith, (Eds.), *The structure of phonological representations. Part II* (pp. 27–68). Dordrecht: Foris.

Ewen, C. (1982b). The phonological representation of the Welsh mutations. In J. Anderson (Ed.), *Language form and linguistic variation* (pp. 80–92). Amsterdam: John Benjamins.

Ewen, C. (1995). Dependency relations in phonology. In J. Goldsmith (Ed.), *The handbook of phonological theory* (pp. 570–585). Oxford: Blackwell.

Ewen, C., & Hulst H. van der (1988). [high], [low] and [back], or [I], [A], and [U]. In P. Coopmans & A. Hulk (Eds.), *Linguistics in the Netherlands 1988* (pp. 51–60). Dordrecht: Foris.

Goldsmith, J. (1993). *The last phonological rule.* Chicago: University of Chicago Press.

Grunwell, P. (1986). *Clinical phonology,* 2nd ed. London: Croom Helm.

Harris, J. (1990). Segmental complexity and phonological government. *Phonology, 7,* 255–300.

Harris, J. (1994). *English sound structure.* Oxford: Blackwell.

Harris, J., & Lindsey, G. (1995). The elements of phonological representation. In J. Durand & F. Katamba (Eds.), *Frontiers of phonology* (pp. 34–79). London: Longmans.

Harrison, P. (1996, May). *The acquisition of melodic primes in infancy.* Paper presented at the 4th Phonology Meeting, University of Manchester.

Hulst, H. van der (1989). Atoms of segmental structure: Components, gestures and dependency. *Phonology, 6,* 253–284.

Hulst, H. van der (1993). *Principles of radical CV phonology.* Manuscript. University of Leiden.

Hulst, H. van der (1994). Radical cv phonology: The locational gesture. *UCL Papers in Linguistics, 6,* 439–478.

Hulst, H. van der (1995). Radical cv phonology: The categorial gesture. In J. Durand & F. Katamba (Eds.), *Frontiers of phonology* (pp. 80–116). London: Longmans.

Hulst, H. van der (1996, May). *Symmetry in phonology.* Paper presented at the 4th Phonology Meeting, University of Manchester.

Hulst, H. van der, & Weijer, J. van de (1995). Non-linear phonology 1982–1994. In H. van der Hulst & J. van de Weijer (Eds.), *Leiden in last* (pp. 1–24). The Hague: Holland Academic Graphics.

Jakobson, R., Fant, G., & Halle, M. (1952). *Preliminaries to speech analysis.* Cambridge, MA: MIT Press.

Jakobson, R., & Halle, M. (1956). *Fundamentals of language.* The Hague: Mouton.

Kaye, J. (1995). Derivations and interfaces. In J. Durand & F. Katamba (Eds.), *Frontiers of phonology* (pp. 289–332). London: Longmans.

Kaye, J., Lowenstamm, J., & Vergnaud, J.-R. (1985). The internal structure of phonological elements: A theory of charm and government. *Phonology Yearbook, 2,* 305–328.

Kaye, J., Lowenstamm, J., & Vergnaud, J.-R. (1990). Constituent structure and government in phonology. *Phonology, 7,* 193–232.

Ladefoged, P. (1971). *Preliminaries to linguistic phonetics.* Chicago: University of Chicago Press.

Ladefoged, P., & Traill, A. (1984). Linguistic phonetic descriptions of clicks. *Language, 60,* 1–20.

Lass, R. (1984). *Phonology.* Cambridge, England: Cambridge University Press.

Levelt, C. (1994). *On the acquisition of place.* The Hague: Holland Academic

Graphics.

Ohala, J. J. (1992). The segment: Primitive or derived? In G. Docherty & R. Ladd (Eds.), *Papers in laboratory phonology II. Gesture, segment, prosody* (pp. 166–183). Cambridge, England: Cambridge University Press.

Ritter, N. (1996, May). *An alternative means of expressing manner.* Paper presented at the 4th Phonology Meeting, University of Manchester.

Roca, I. (1994). *Generative phonology.* London: Routledge.

Sagey, E. (1986). *The representation of features and relations in non-linear phonology.* Ph.D. Dissertation, Massachusetts Institute of Technology.

Schane, S. (1995). Diphthongization in particle phonology. In J. Goldsmith (Ed.), *The handbook of phonological theory* (pp. 586–608). Oxford: Blackwell.

Trubetzkoy, N. (1969 [original 1939]). *Principles of phonology.* Berkeley: University of California Press.

CHAPTER

Grounded Phonology: Application to the Analysis of Disordered Speech

BARBARA HANDFORD BERHARDT
CAROL STOEL-GAMMON

This chapter provides an overview of Archangeli and Pulleyblank's (1994) theory presented in their book *Grounded Phonology*, and extends and applies major concepts of that work to analysis of child phonology. The main proposals of *Grounded Phonology* concern underlying representation of phonological form (Combinatorial Specification), the relationship between phonetics and phonology (phonetic *grounding* of phonological phenomena), and phonological rule parameterization. Because of space limitations, we focus primarily on the application of Combinatorial Specification in this chapter, presenting an analysis and intervention plan for a child with a severe phonological disorder. The concept of phonetic grounding is described briefly in terms of cleft palate speech, and also during the case discussion where applicable. Throughout the chapter, basic concepts of nonlinear phonological theory are employed, including hierarchical syllable and word structure and feature geometry. (See also Bernhardt & Stoel-Gammon, 1994; Dinnsen, Chapter 4; Ingram, Chapter 2.)

In the first part of the chapter, we introduce Combinatorial Specification, phonetic grounding, and rule parameterization. In the second part of the chapter, we contrast phonological process and Combinatorial Specification analyses for one child with a phonological disorder (DE, from Stoel-Gammon & Dunn, 1985), showing the utility of the theory of Combinatorial Specification for explaining patterns observed and setting goals for intervention.

GROUNDED PHONOLOGY: THEORETICAL CONCEPTS

Combinatorial Specification

Combinatorial Specification is a theory about phonological representation; features, features values, and feature combinations are the primitives of this theory. Some features and values are considered to be stored in underlying representation, whereas other system-redundant features and values are assumed to be "filled in" automatically during speech processing. We first provide a historical background of feature theory, and then describe key concepts of Combinatorial Specification, namely:

1. Primitives of the theory: F-elements (feature values) and feature associations
2. Feature combinations (alternately, "paths")
3. Status of feature values: default, redundant, or specified
4. Universal defaults versus language- or child-specific defaults

Extensions of the theory of Combinatorial Specification, such as Default Underspecification (see Bernhardt & Stemberger, in press), and Context-Sensitive Underspecification (Dinnsen, 1996) are also briefly discussed.

Historical Background

Generative phonology has long been concerned with characterization of speech sounds (segments) in terms of distinctive features. Feature theory has responded to three major observations:

1. Individual speech sounds may share certain phonetic properties.
2. Languages (and child phonological systems) have different segmental inventories.
3. Some speech sounds are more frequent than others crosslinguistically and in child speech.

By positing units smaller than the segment, generalizations about similarities and differences among segments within and across languages can be captured. In early versions of distinctive feature theory, features were considered inherent properties of segments, or phonemes (Jakobson, Fant, & Halle, 1963). Feature values were assumed to be binary: a feature was either present ([+]) or not present ([−]). Segments, features, and values that occur frequently across languages and in child phonology were considered to be **unmarked** and less frequent ones more **marked**. Chomsky and Halle (1968) followed generally in the earlier tradition, but alternatively proposed that features were not properties of segments but, rather, segments were composed of bundles of features. In other words, segments were derivatives of features. Each segment was assumed to have underlying values for all features (full specification), although presence of some features and values implied the presence of others, through what Chomsky and Halle (1968) called markedness conventions.

In trying to account for the difference in frequency of occurrence among features and the consequences for phonological patterns, some phonologists in the 1980s began to question the concept of full underlying specification. Variants of the theory of **underspecification** were proposed; these assume minimal storage of feature information in underlying representation. During speech production processing, some feature content is automatically supplied for output because of built-in redundancies in the phonological system. The two main variants of underspecification of the 1980s were Contrastive Specification (e.g., Clements, 1987; Steriade, 1987) and Radical Underspecification (e.g., Archangeli, 1988; Kiparsky, 1982; Pulleyblank, 1986). Both of these theories continue to assume the derivative notion of segment. However, Contrastive Specification assumes that feature specifications are stored in underlying representation when needed to contrast segments, whereas Radical Underspecification assumes that underlying representations include only unpredictable values for features characterizing the segments of an inventory. In both theories, predictable values are assumed to be inserted by redundancy rules during output processing.

Combinatorial Specification has much in common with Radical Underspecification in terms of the concepts of minimal specification, and lack of the relevance of contrast. The segment (phoneme) has no status in Combinatorial Specification, however. Archangeli and Pulleyblank draw attention to the fact that feature combinations (paths) occur at single discrete points in time (as in a segment) but note that features can be linked over several timing units (1994, pp. 44–46). For example, in English, the feature [+nasal] can spread from a consonant to the preceding vowel. The vowel is not a "nasal" vowel per se, but is produced with nasality because of the adjacent nasal consonant. Thus, they claim that segments are neither primitives of the system, nor necessarily discrete units. Other differences between Radical Underspecification and Combinatorial Specification relate to markedness and underlying representation; we elaborate that discussion below.

"F"-elements in Combinatorial Specification

"F-elements" are primitive units of representation in Combinatorial Specification. This term refers to features (such as [voice]), feature values ([+voice] versus [–voice]), and class nodes of the feature geometry (such as Root, Laryngeal, or Place nodes). Class (or organizing) nodes have no feature content themselves, but denote groups of features that pattern together phonologically, as proposed in most accounts of feature geometry. Appendix 6–1 gives features of adult English that have specified (nondefault) [+] or [–] values, plus the class or organizing nodes. In accordance with general principles of nonlinear phonology, each feature is considered to have independent (autosegmental) status in the geometry. However, realization of a particular feature crucially depends on its association (time-based link, or combination) with other features. Not all combinations occur, either because of the relationships within the feature hierarchy, or because of the language itself (or the child's system, in our case). We return to issues regarding feature combination after a discussion of feature values and specification.

Status of Feature Values

As noted, only unpredictable features and feature values are present in underlying representation. Predictable features or feature values appearing in surface forms but not present in underlying representation are inserted during the course of the derivation. (Archangeli & Pulleyblank note that not all redundant features may be inserted during processing, but only those definitely needed for articulation [1994, p. 60]).

What is meant by specified (unpredictable) versus redundant (predictable, or default) feature value? There appear to be two types of redundancy: those that are inherent in the definition of features themselves and those that are particular to a language or child's system. To illustrate, we provide a discussion of the feature [sonorant] and its relationship to [voice] and [spread glottis]. These features exemplify apparent conundrums in underspecification. Laryngeal features are also particularly significant for the case example we describe later in the chapter.

Typically, sonorants (vowels, glides, nasals, liquids) are voiced, the state of the vocal folds allowing spontaneous voicing (Chomsky & Halle, 1968; Rice, 1993).

(1) [+sonorant] IMPLIES >> [+voice], or Spontaneous Voicing (SV)

(Rice, 1993, actually renames [sonorant] as Spontaneous Voicing (SV) and gives this feature status as a class node similar to Place.) Sonorants may be produced without voicing (e.g., voiceless nasals). Lombardi (1991) and Mester and Itô (1989) suggest that such voiceless sonorants are produced with a spread glottis. Spontaneous voicing for sonorants does not occur when the glottis is spread, although there are languages with highly marked, breathy voiced obstruents ("murmur" in Hindi). Thus:

(2) [+spread glottis] IMPLIES >> [–voice]

The feature [+spread glottis] is considered to be underlying for voiceless resonants, for /h/, and for word-initial aspirated stops in English (see Appendix 6–1). Thus, we have a case where redundancies are not always the same: [+sonorant] usually implies [+voice], but if it occurs in combination with [+spread glottis], it does not imply [+voice] because of the phonetic incompatibility of a spread glottis and spontaneous voicing.

Another apparent paradox exists with respect to [sonorant] and [voice]. Stops and fricatives, which are [–sonorant], can be produced with voicing. Thus, [–sonorant] does not necessarily imply [–voice], although crosslinguistically, voiceless obstruents are more common than voiced obstruents (Maddieson, 1984). Thus, according to Radical Underspecification and Combinatorial Specification, the feature [–voice] is generally considered the system default (underspecified) value for obstruents.

(3)   [0voice] IMPLIES >> [–voice]

For languages that have only voiceless obstruents (contrasting with voiced sonorants), specification of [voice] is completely redundant and determined by implication: [+sonorant] implies [+voice] and [–sonorant] implies [–voice]. Designation of default features becomes more complex, however, when languages have both voiced and unvoiced obstruents. If [+voice] is redundant for sonorants, how can the same feature value ([+voice]) be the nondefault value for obstruents? Several explanations have been given for this paradox. Chomsky and Halle (1968) and others more recently (e.g., McCarthy & Prince, 1993) argue that such cases show the need for full specification. Bernhardt and Stemberger (in press) present a variant of underspecification theory called Default Underspecification, in which there are two kinds of redundant features: those presumed by phonetically grounded cooccurrence restrictions such as the [+spread glottis]-[–voice] case, and those that arise in a particular grammar (system defaults). (See Appendix 6–3.) This is in essence an extension of Archangeli and Pulleyblank's (1994) view that, although there are universal trends for defaults/specified features, individual grammars may have underlying specification for some features that are typically defaults in others.

Another variable aspect of underspecification is discussed by Dinnsen (1996) who suggests that underspecification may show context sensitivity; that is, underspecified values may differ for different word positions. Archangeli and Pulleyblank (1994) do not adopt this point of view, but it adds another possible dimension to underspecification theory. We consider its relevance in the data section of this chapter.

Status of features as binary or privative (unary) is also an issue for feature specification. In earlier versions of feature theory, features were usually considered binary (although Trubetzkoy [1939/1969] noted that some features could be privative or equipollent). Subsequently, some theorists have taken the position that all features are privative. Avery and Rice (1989) suggest that features are either present ([+F]) or completely absent ([0F]). Other phonologists (e.g., Sagey, 1986) have assumed that some features are privative, in particular, the class nodes (Root, Place, Laryngeal) and place features ([Labial], [Coronal], [Dorsal]), but that others are binary. Terminal features of the geometry are considered binary in such versions of the theory. Combinatorial Specification is essentially neutral with respect to the issue of binarity. The focus of Combinatorial Specification is the combination of features, each combination having its own set of conditions that can override individual features or feature values. Archangeli and Pulleyblank (1994) suggest that setting up a theory in terms of feature value designation may potentially lead to the wrong set of predictions relative to conditions on combinations. Thus, Combinatorial Specification starts with the more demanding set of conditions, those concerning combination.

Universal, Language- or Child-specific Defaults

Combinatorial Specification differs from previous theories of underspecification in terms of predictions about which features and feature values are likely to be underlying versus redundant. According to Radical Underspecification, the default (redundancy) rules correspond to universal markedness considerations (Archangeli, 1988, p. 197). However, examination of vowel data sets from different languages led Archangeli and Pulleyblank (1994) to the observation that, although there are trends across languages, different languages can have different underspecified values for features. Combinatorial Specification allows supposedly "universally unmarked" (predictable) features or values to be specified in underlying representation in some languages. Although this type of powerful flexibility may appear to be a weakness of their theory, it has appeal in terms of child phonology. It has long been noted that in spite of common patterns in phonological acquisition, there is also a considerable degree of variation across children with both typical and disordered phonological development (Grunwell, 1985; Macken & Ferguson, 1983). Acquisition patterns for manner of articulation appear fairly strong: Most children produce stops and nasals early in development, and fricatives and liquids later, suggesting that the feature [−continuant] is a default consonant feature from early on, whereas [+continuant] is a nondefault consonant feature that has to be learned. Place features, on the other hand, show more variation. For example, many children may have the universally expected coronal default (Stemberger & Stoel-Gammon, 1991). However, some children have a labial place default (using only labial consonants in early phonology), and others have a strong velar preference (Menn, 1975; Stoel-Gammon & Cooper, 1984). (See Bernhardt & Stoel-Gammon, 1996, for a more complete discussion of acquisition versus universal defaults.)

Classification of features as default or specified is not a straightforward task. Archangeli and Pulleyblank (1994) have developed their theory through an in-depth examination of crosslinguistic patterns for only one feature, [ATR] (Advanced Tongue Root). Detailed studies of each language and its particular patterns (in our case, of each child's phonological patterns) are needed to determine the probable status of features, as defaults or nondefaults (specified). We give our assumptions for full and underspecified features of English consonants in Appendixes 6–1 and 6–2.

Feature Combinations (Paths) in Combinatorial Specification

As noted previously, features can only be produced in combination with other features. Thus, links between features are also primitives of representation, according to Combinatorial Specification. Feature links can occur simultaneously (the [Labial] and [–continuant] features of /p/), or can occur over timing units (when features "spread" between units). Links are expressed formally with association lines. When features are linked with other features, they are said to be "on a path" with those features. Some features may be present in underlying representation, but not necessarily be represented in combination with other features. Tone features or features of epenthetic segments are sometimes in this situation as "floating" features, which surface when words require them. Not all combinations of features are possible. One of the challenges of phonological theory is to account for possible and impossible feature combinations. One of the main purposes of **grounded phonology** is to determine conditions for feature cooccurrence, discussed in the next section.

Grounding Conditions

Not all feature combinations occur across or within languages. Some constraints on feature combination are formal or logical: for example, cooccurrence of [–F] and [+F] is highly improbable, because [+] and [–] are opposites. Others are substantive; for example, combinations may be precluded or promoted because of phonetically grounded constraints on output. Thus, nasals are typically voiced; hence the presence of [+nasal] precludes the presence of [–voice] and the presence of [+nasal] implies [+voice]. Feature status as a default or nondefault can also affect patterns of feature combination, as we will see in the case study description.

In the section on defaults, we noted that markedness and specification are not necessarily considered interdependent according to Combinatorial Specification. However, the notion of markedness is still very much part of Archangeli and Pulleyblank's (1994) theory. The **"Grounding Hypothesis"** is invoked as a way of constraining feature combinations, and as such, incorporates the notion of markedness. The Grounding Hypothesis states that combinations of F-elements are restricted by conditions whose content is closely governed by phonetic properties. The stronger a phonetic implication, the greater its role in determining segmental inventories and relative markedness of different inventories. Two "grounding conditions" are described in the book:

I. Path conditions invoked by languages must be phonetically motivated.
II. The stronger the phonetic motivation for a path condition Φ,
   a. the greater the likelihood of invoking Φ,
   b. the greater the likelihood of assigning a wide scope to Φ within a grammar.
And vice versa.

Archangeli & Pulleyblank, 1994, p. 177

The first condition is an absolute condition. To some degree, the combination of phonological features must have a phonetic basis. For example, given a normal oral mechanism, [–nasal] cannot cooccur with [+nasal], because the velar port is either open (giving [+nasal]) or closed (giving [–nasal]).

The second condition allows for relativity in phonetic motivation. As we noted earlier, sonorants can be either voiced or voiceless. Thus, it is phonetically possible for [+nasal] to combine with [+voice] or [–voice], as per condition I. However, the combination of [+nasal] and [+voice] has a stronger phonetic motivation, because spontaneous voicing of sonorants is more likely, as per condition II.

These conditions apply both to acoustic and articulatory parameters for speech, in other words, to speech perception as well as production. In terms of children's speech, Archangeli and Pulleyblank suggest that a learner's initial hypotheses will reflect physically motivated conditions. Both perceptual conditions (acoustic) and oral mechanism maturity can then affect speech production.

In terms of disordered speech, we may assume that hearing impairment or abnormalities in vocal tracts may have an even stronger effect on phonetic grounding for feature combinations. Given normal hearing and a normal vocal tract, the typical consonant is produced with oral airstream only. The redundant value for the feature [nasal] is [–nasal]. Consonants /m/, /n/, or /ŋ/, are, in contrast, underlying specified as [+nasal]. However, if a person cannot perceive the distinction between nasal and nonnasal resonance, or if the velar port can be only partially occluded as in the case of a cleft palate, speech sounds are typically produced with nasal airflow (i.e., [+nasal]), e.g., /b/ > [m]), or with both oral and nasal airflow ([−nasal] and [+nasal], yielding a nasalized [b̃]).

If a speaker is conscious of the failed attempts to produce a nonnasal segment, we can assume that this person's underlying values for the feature [nasal] are the same as those of people with normal mechanisms. If the deficiency in the perceptual or oral mechanisms can be corrected through auditory amplification (for hearing loss), surgery, or palatal appliances (for cleft palate), a person with an intact phonological system can then adapt quickly to the normalized mechanism(s). Speech sounds will be produced accurately, because of the already correct phonological values for the feature [nasal]. The problem for such a person is in actual articulatory implementation, not in phonological representation or processing. However, some speakers continue to produce nonnasal target segments with nasal airflow, even after surgical and/or other therapeutic interventions. In such cases, these speakers may have different phonological default values and assumptions about possible feature combinations. The feature value [+nasal] may be the default value phonologically, and combinations of [+nasal] and [−nasal] may be considered legitimate. Speech intervention in this case needs to address both the phonological and articulatory levels with therapy focusing on the contrast between oral and nasal airflow, and the phonological fact that most speech sounds are oral (i.e., the default value for [nasal] is [−nasal]). (For further discussion of the application of Combinatorial Specification to the description of cleft palate speech, see Bernhardt, Doan, & Stoel-Gammon, 1995.)

Bernhardt and Stemberger (in press) suggest that phonetic grounding is not the only type of grounding for feature combinations and phonological patterns. Cognitive and processing resources may also limit the output potential. Many children with phonological disorders appear to have no abnormalities in their perception of speech or in their oral mechanisms. In these cases, it may be that cognitive or processing variables may be particularly constraining. For a child whose segmental output is affected by relative complexity and resource limitations, combinations of nondefault (specified) features may be less likely than combinations involving default features. For example, a child may be able to produce [p] and [s], but not [f]. In terms of feature specification, we can assume that [p] has a specified [Labial] feature plus default manner and voice features, [−continuant] and [−voice], and that [s] has a specified manner feature, [+continuant], and default place feature, [Coronal]. In terms of feature complexity, [p] and [s] are therefore equivalent. On the other hand, [f] is more complex in terms of specification. It has two nondefault features, [labial] and [+continuant]. Production of a segment with more stored features such as [f] could be seen to require more cognitive resources. Thus, cognitive limitations can also potentially constrain speech output.

Before leaving this discussion, we note that many speakers are able to compensate for aberrant mechanisms and maintain the phonological contrasts for their language. Speakers with unrepaired cleft palates may completely distinguish between various sound classes through use of what parts of the mechanism are functioning. Thus, pharyngeal, glottal, and palatal stops as well as fricatives, nasals, and laterally released segments may replace a variety of target consonants in a way that remains contrastive (Howard, 1993). Furthermore, some speakers are able to produce reasonable phonetic variants of the target sounds, even if the mechanism does not function in the expected way (Dworkin & Culatta, 1985). In such cases, cognitive resources are recruited to overcome phonetic constraints. We remarked above that some children have normal mechanisms (for their age) and yet have phonological disorders. Thus, the interplay between phonetic and cognitive grounding of constraints is important to consider for a given individual.

We have framed the previous discussion in terms of constraints rather than rules or processes. Because phonological theory in the past 40 years has described phonological patterns in terms of rules or processes affecting underlying representations, we will outline Archangeli and Pulleyblank's (1994) framework for rule parameterization in the next section because rules or processes can be useful descriptors for the patterns observed. In the case study that follows, we present first a processes analysis of his data, and then assume constraints for the nonlinear phonological description.

Phonological Rule Parameters

Archangeli and Pulleyblank (1994) outline four types of parameters relative to phonological rules.

1. Rule function: insertion or deletion
2. Type: path or F-element
3. Directionality
4. Iterativity

Insertion and Deletion of Features or Feature Values

According to Archangeli and Pulleyblank (1994), phonological operations involve insertion and/or deletion of phonological information.
These can affect prosodic structure units, features, or feature values.
Insertion results in creation of new links (association lines) between
phonological elements, whereas deletion results in delinking of elements (removal of association lines between them). Features may be
prohibited (a) everywhere in a system (b) only in combination with
other features, or (c) only in certain word positions. We give examples
from child phonology as a background for the case study that follows.

Consider first an example with a privative (nonbinary) feature,
such as a place feature. If a child cannot produce velars, (whether in all
or some word positions), the feature [Dorsal] must be deleted and
some other feature must be inserted in place of [dorsal]. Typically, children "front" velars, that is, produce alveolar segments in their place
(Stoel-Gammon, 1996). In such cases, the default place feature [coro-
nal] is linked up (inserted). Note that only the place feature is affected.
The manner and voice features are inserted as they would be for the
target velar. Thus, /k/ is produced as [t], /g/ as [d], and /ŋ/ as [n],
given that no other processes or constraints are operative.

Rules affecting binary features operate similarly. The underlying
feature values may be deleted, and redundant values inserted. For
example, if a child produces a /b/ as a [p], the underlying feature
[+voice] is delinked, and [–voice] is inserted. The place and manner
features of /b/ do not change since /b/ and [p] are both [Labial] and
[–continuant].

Sometimes, features can only occur in certain combinations and not
others, as we noted above in the discussion of cognitive grounding. For
example, /f/ has two specified features, [Labial] and [+continuant]. If a
child cannot produce a segment with two specified features, one option
is to delink one of the specified features and insert a default feature for
that particular feature (as we showed for [Coronal]). If [+continuant] is
deleted, /f/ will surface as [p]. If, however, [Labial] is deleted, the segment is unspecified then for place. The default place [Coronal] will be
then inserted by redundancy rules, /f/ surfacing as [s].

Directionality

Directionality of rules goes beyond restrictions on a particular feature
or feature combinations and concerns relationships of one segment to
another. In child phonology, directionality of rules is seen primarily in

terms of assimilation (spreading of features). A child may show evidence of regressive assimilation ([gʌk] for *duck)* but no progressive assimilation, for example, *[kʌk] is never produced for *cut*. In such cases, the velar assimilation rule (spread of the feature [Dorsal]) applies from right-to-left, but not from left-to-right (see Stoel-Gammon, 1996, for examples).

Iterativity

Iterativity also refers to more than one segment in a word. A child may show evidence of assimilation on all segments of a word, or only on some. For example, Harry (Stemberger & Bernhardt, Chapter 7), showed iterative assimilation, but iterativity was limited so that onsets of syllables with primary stress (before compounding) remained impervious to the spreading process. (Furthermore, the number of links could be no more than a multiple of two.) For example:

(4) television   /tɛləvɪʒən/   ['tɛ-nəninən] (2^2)
musicbox   /mjuzɪk#baks/   [mumi-(#')ta] (2^1)
(# is a word boundary marker.)

We turn now to a case study demonstrating the application of concepts of Combinatorial Specification to disordered speech, both for analysis and for selecting goals for intervention.

APPLICATION OF GROUNDED PHONOLOGY TO ANALYSIS OF PHONOLOGICALLY DISORDERED SPEECH

This section provides analyses of a speech sample from a child with a phonological disorder to demonstrate the utility of the theory of Combinatorial Specification. First, as background for that discussion, we present more familiar analyses based on those procedures: phonetic and word shape inventories, match and substitution analyses, and phonological process analysis (see Stoel-Gammon & Dunn, 1985, Chapter 6). The inventory and substitution analyses provide a basis for the combinatorial feature analysis which follows. The Combinatorial Specification analysis will be shown to account for some of the patterns designated as variable or inconsistent in the other approaches and to serve as a basis for selection of more precise goals for treatment.

Traditional Phonological Analyses

General Subject Description

DE (Stoel-Gammon & Dunn, 1985) was reported to have highly unintelligible speech. Based on a 91-word sample of single- and two-word utterances at age 4;6, his percentage consonants correct was 43% (a moderately severe disorder, according to Shriberg & Kwiatkowski, 1982). Vowels, although not 100% accurate, were not considered sufficiently disordered to warrant treatment. (See Stoel-Gammon & Dunn, 1985, p. 144, for the complete data set.) At assessment, the following additional factors were noted:

1. Normal hearing according to a hearing screening (with a history of otitis media);
2. An apparent normal oral mechanism (although he was unwilling to tolerate a comprehensive oral mechanism examination); and
3. A possible delay in language comprehension and production (although he was reluctant to speak in the testing situation, and hence this could not be reliably determined).

Syllable and Word Structure: Inventory and Match Data

Words generally had the same number of syllables as the adult target. Only two words of the assessment sample were reduced in length (*television* was produced as [tsɛzɪn], *hanger* as [hʌ̃n]). However, in terms of CV configurations, 42 words (46%) were simplified in comparison with the adult target. The major word shape restriction involved clusters for which there were 40 targets and only 8 matches (8/40 matches: 20%). DE displayed more difficulty for onset and coda clusters than for medial heterosyllabic consonant sequences (C.C, where the period indicates a syllable boundary). Key characteristics of word and syllable structure based on an independent analysis of word and syllable shape inventories were:

1. Most frequent word shapes: CVC (38) and CVCV (13)
2. Maximum word length of the sample: Three syllables in *screwdriver*: [ʃudaɪbɚ]
3. Word-initial clusters: 5/22 targets: [sw] (3, in *spring, string, squirrel*), [tʃw] in *quarter*, [fl] in *flower*
4. Word-final clusters: 1/4 targets: [zd] in *closed*
5. Medial onset clusters: 0/3 targets

6. Word-internal consonant sequences in CVCCVC words: 5/8 targets ([tm] in *Christmas*, [sr] in *toothbrush*, [nd] in *candle* and *finger*, [tb] in *football*, but not [lg], [sb], or [sk] in *Fall Guy*, *baseball*, or *basket*).

In summary, DE's sample is characterized by relative breadth in syllable/word shapes. He produced open and closed syllables, multisyllabic forms, and a few consonant clusters ([sw-], [tʃw-], [fl-], [-zd]).

Phonetic Consonantal Inventory

DE's phonetic inventory by word position appears in Table 6–1. Present in the inventory (independent of whether they matched adult targets) were:

1. Segments representing all manner classes across all word positions: stops, nasals, glides, fricatives, affricates, liquids
2. Labial and Coronal place segments in all word positions
3. Two non-English word-initial segments, [ts] (5 tokens), and [ʒ] (one token)
4. Alveopalatals: [ʃ] (3 tokens), [tʃ] and [ʒ] (once each as word-initial substitutions)
5. Three word-initial cluster types, [sw], [tʃw], and [fl], and one word-final cluster, [zd].

Consonant Matches and Substitution Patterns

In word-initial and word-final positions, 52% of DE's consonants matched adult targets, whereas only 32% matched adult targets in medial positions (onset and coda). Consistent matches with adult targets were found for:

1. The glide /w/
2. Labial and Coronal nasals and voiced stops: /m/, /n/, /b/, /d/
3. Voicing
4. Clusters /fl/ and /zd/

Inconsistent matches were noted across word positions for:

1. Labiodental fricatives /f/ and /v/
2. The unvoiced stops /p/ and /t/
3. Coronal alveolar fricatives /s/ and /z/

Table 6–1. Consonant matches, substitutions, and deletions.

Adult Target	Word-initial	Medial Onset	Medial Coda	Word-final
m	✓ (4)	✓		✓
mj	m			
mp				p
n	✓ (2)	✓ (2)	✓ (2)	✓ (9)
nd				ø, n
ndʒ				d
ŋ			n (2)	n (2)
p	s, f	✓, t, f		✓ (4)
pl		s		
b	✓ (5)	✓ (3)		✓
br	b	r		
t	✓, s (2), ts (2), z	✓ (3), ø (1)	✓	✓ (2)
tr	tʰ			
ts				z
d	✓			✓ (2)
dr		d		
k	s (5), ts	t, d, ø		t (6), ø (1)
kl	s (3)			
kw	tʃw			
g	z	d		d
gl	s (2), z			
gr	w, s			
f	✓ (3), s (3), ts	s		✓ (3)
fl	✓			
v	b	✓, b, ø		z
θ	z		s	f
θr	tʰ, r			
ð	d	d		
s	✓ (2)	z	✓, t, ø	✓ (3), ts
sp	s			
st	tʰ, s			
sk	z			

continued

Adult Target	Word-initial	Medial Onset	Medial Coda	Word-final
sn	s			
sl	s			
spr	sw			
str	sw			
skw	sw			
skr	∫			
z	✓	s		✓ (5)
zd				✓
∫	✓, s			✓, s
ʒ		z		
t∫	s			ts (2)
dʒ	d, ʒ			ts
r	✓ (2), w (2)	z	✓ (1), ø (1)	✓ (4), V (11), ø (3)ᵃ
l	✓, s, z	ø (2), z	ø (1)	✓ (2), ø (2), ʌ
w	✓ (2)			
j	✓, ts	✓		
h	✓ (2), ø (2)			

Note: If no number given, assume 1 token; ✓ indicates correct production.
ᵃ This category includes vocalic /r/ and final /r/ clusters. V indicates vowel.

4. Glides and liquids /h/, /j/, /l/ and /r/
5. Alveolpalatals /∫/, /t∫/, and /ʒ/

Completely absent from the phonetic inventory sample were:

1. Dorsal place consonants (velars)
2. Interdentals [θ] and [ð]
3. The voiced alveolpalatal [dʒ]
4. Word-initial [p] and [v], and word-final [v]
5. All clusters except /fl/ and /zd/

Common substitutions were:

1. Coronal (alveolar) fricatives [s] and [z], or the affricate [ts], appearing for target fricatives, stops, liquids, and /j/ in onsets (primarily in word-initial onset)

2. Coronal stops, as substitutions for fricatives or velar stops in non-word-initial positions (5 times)
3. The cluster [sw], appearing for /skw/, /str/, and /spr/, and the cluster [tʃw], appearing for /kw/

DE thus showed use of a variety of segments, with notable exceptions being velars, interdentals, and certain labials. Substitution patterns were relatively common in some cases (alveolars for velars) and rare in others (alveolar fricatives or affricates appearing for other fricatives, stops or approximants, particularly word initially).

Intervention Goal Selection: Inventory and Substitution Analysis

Before distinctive feature analysis and phonological process analysis became utilized in articulation/phonological therapy, segmental inventory and substitution analyses provided the basis for setting goals in intervention. Segments were targeted one at a time, starting with sounds that are acquired early developmentally, according to available norms. Often, "stimulable" phones were selected as targets, but not necessarily. In DE's case, a developmental and stimulability approach could result in the following goal sequence:

1. Inconsistent early-acquired segments: /p/, /t/, and /h/
2. Later-acquired segments: Velars, /f/
3. Latest-acquired segments: Other fricatives and liquids, clusters (order to be determined by the particular set of developmental norms being followed and relative stimulability).

If only absent sounds were targeted, velars, /dʒ/, /θ/, and /ð/ and clusters would be targeted in approximately that order.

Although a remediation program can be constructed on the basis of developmental norms and segmental inventories, there are three problems with this approach: (a) the lack of reliable norms upon which to project reasonable goals; (b) the variability across children in order of acquisition, making even reliable norms irrelevant in the case of an individual child; and (c) the lack of generalization in treatment, resulting in long periods of therapy. In the 1970s, speech-language pathology adopted methodologies used by linguists to analyze phonological samples. The child's (mis)pronunciations were no longer viewed as sound-by-sound deviations from the adult target, but as systematic, rule-governed productions. Both distinctive feature analysis (e.g., Compton, 1970; Oller, 1973) and phonological process analysis came into clinical use (Edwards & Bernhardt, 1973; Grunwell, 1985; Hodson & Paden, 1983, 1991). Phonological process analysis gained wider acceptance in clinical application, probably because it described not only segmental changes and patterns, but also word and syllable structure changes and patterns in a child's speech. Thus we focus on phonological process analysis only in the next section. How do the observations and goals derived from inventory analyses compare with process analysis results?

Phonological Process Analysis

Phonological processes are listed in Table 6–2, based primarily on analyses generated by the Interactive System for Phonological Analysis (Masterson & Pagan, 1993). The major processes were as follows:

1. Syllable structure: Cluster Reduction (83%).
2. Substitution processes (occurring at least 40% of the time according to opportunity for occurrence):
   a. Velar Fronting (82%, including use of [s] for /k/ or /g/)
   b. Depalatalization (50%)
   c. Deaffrication (57%)
3. Spirantization, Affrication, Fricative and Alveolar Assimilation: frequent processes but incalculable due to overlap among processes.

The segments [s], [z], and [ts] were frequent word-initial substitutions. A number of possible substitution and assimilation processes could result in these substitutions. For example, compare *couch, two* and *yellow* in terms of Affrication versus Alveolar Assimilation:

(5) yellow   /jɛloʊ/   [tsaʊ]
    two   /tu:/   [tsʊ]
    couch   /kaʊtʃ/   [tsaʊts]

The [ts] substitution appears for /t/, /j/ and /k/. In the first two cases, it appears to be Affrication of coronal segments. In *couch*, we could also call it affrication, but usually word-initial /k/ appears as [s]. Hence, there is a possibility of assimilation between the onset and coda because of the final affricate. In DE's sample, affrication can occur independently, but is more likely when there is already an affricate in the word. Calculating frequency of occurrence and opportunities for oc-

Table 6–2. Phonological processes for DE's sample.

Phonological Process	Number of Opportunities	Frequency (in %)	Targets Affected
Syllable Structure			
Segment Deletion			
Initial position	60	3	/h/
Medial onset	30	17	/k, ʃ, r, l/
Medial coda	10	30	/s, l/
Final	52	6	/k, l/
Weak syllable deletion	35	6	Medial and final syllables
Cluster reduction	40	83	All
Substitution			
Velar fronting	38	82	All positions
Stopping	62	13	All fricatives, I affricate
Depalatalization	16	50	Initial, final
Gliding	32	16	Initial, medial onset
Vocalization	28	36	Final
Deaffrication	7	57	Initial, (Final: I time)
Palatalization	2 **actual** occ	a	Initial /kw/: [tʃw] Initial /skr/: [ʃ]
Spirantization	13 **actual** occ	a	Initial, medial onset
Affrication	6 **actual** occ	a	Initial
Assimilation	**Number of Actual Occurrences**		
Fricative	11	b	Initial
Coronal (alveolar)	22	b	Initial

a = Potential occurrences and percentage of occurrence were not identified because these processes interacted with fricative and alveolar assimilation processes.

b = Fricative assimilation was counted whenever a nonfricative was produced as fricative in the presence of another fricative. Alveolar assimilation was counted whenever a nonalveolar was produced as an alveolar in the presence of another alveolar.

currence becomes very difficult with these types of interactions among process types.

Process analysis indicates a moderate degree of variability in the data (as does substitution analysis). Variability occurs across segment type, word position, and for the same word. Note that even in the quantifiable processes listed above, none occurred 100% of the time. In general, more processes appear to affect word-initial position. Processes sometimes were different for the same segment, depending on word position. For example, velars were fronted to alveolar fricatives in word-initial position, but to alveolar stops in other positions.

(6)   gun   /gʌn/   [zʌn]
      Fall Guy   /fɑl#gaɪ/   [sʌdaɪ]

Fricatives and affricates were occasionally stopped, but stops /p/ and /t/ were often spirantized or affricated in word-initial position (when they were not aspirated).

(7)   Christmas   /krɪsməs/   [sɪtmʌs]
BUT: toothbrush   /tuθ#brʌʃ/   [tʰusrəʃ]
      page   /peɪdʒ/   [sets]
      ten   /tɛn/   [zɛn] (also see *two* above)

Some fricatives were affricated, but some affricates were deaffricated, with word-initial position again causing the most difficulty.

(8)   ice   /aɪs/   [aɪts]
      chair   /tʃɛr/   [sɛɚ]
      Joe   /dʒoʊ/   [do]
      jump   /dʒʌmp/   [ʒʌp]

Spirantization and Affrication appear to be randomly interchangeable in some cases, and affected by assimilation in others (as we showed above). Deaspiration of word-initial stops and Cluster Reduction are common, but do not always occur. Cluster Reduction can affect one or the other element of a cluster both for the same word, and across words.

(9)   green   /grin/   [wĩn], [sĩn]
      star   /star/   [saʌ]
      stick   /stɪk/   [tʰɪ]

Thus, although we can identify certain types of processes, quantitative analysis is not particularly helpful in analyzing the patterns that occur. Calculation of actual and potential occurrences is compromised by process overlap. Apparent variability may result in lower scores of occurrence for individual processes, yet the variability itself appears to be a relevant factor in the overall system, compromising the pattern analysis described by phonological process analysis.

Intervention Goal Selection: Phonological Process Analysis

Intervention based on pattern analyses such as phonological process analysis is viewed as more efficient than intervention based on segment-by-segment approaches because of the potential for generalization: targeting one representative exemplar of the process may lead to positive changes for other phonemes affected by that process. For example, teaching /k/ may lead to elimination of Velar Fronting on all three velar targets, /k/, /g/, and /ŋ/.

Various approaches exist regarding selection of therapy goals. Generally, it is argued that processes occurring frequently, processes that disappear early in normal development and processes that interfere significantly with speech intelligibility should be targeted first. Grunwell (1985) presents a developmental chart for processes, and suggests targeting those that tend to drop out of normal speech early, but notes also that unusual processes and variability are also important considerations in goal selection. Edwards (Edwards, Bernhardt, & Gierut, 1992) suggests an additional consideration with respect to interdependencies of processes. If one process is dependent on another, the more basic one must be addressed first. For example, if /ʃ/ > [t], but /s/ > [t], it is assumed by rule ordering that /ʃ/ > [s], then [s] > [t]. Thus, /s/ should be trained before /ʃ/.

One cannot rely solely on developmental charts for DE, because his phonology does not appear to be following a typical path in terms of acquisition of consonants in word-initial position. However, according to Grunwell's (1985) six-stage chart, DE would be functioning between Stage IV and V. Major Stage V processes evident in DE's speech were Depalatalization, Stopping of voiced fricatives, Cluster Reduction, and Gliding of liquids. The degree of Cluster Reduction is more typical of Stage IV, however, and Velar Fronting is more typical of Stage III. Thus, Cluster Reduction and Velar Fronting appear to be relevant processes to target in the first therapy period. The Affrication, Deaffrication, Spirantization, and Assimilation processes do not fit into Grunwell's (1985) developmental scheme, but need to be listed as unusual or idiosyncratic processes. Thus, they need to be targeted. The variability, particularly across word position, may suggest a need to target the processes independently by word position. Edwards' suggestion about ordering of processes would lead to targeting velars first in non-word-initial position because, presumably, velars are first fronted, and then spirantized word initially.

(10)   /k/ > [t]
       [t] > [s] or [ts]

First period (cycle) goals based on our interpretation of Grunwell's and Edwards' suggestions would then be:

1. Velar fronting, with targeting of word-initial position prior to other positions.
2. Spirantization/Stopping/Fricative or Alveolar Assimilation (alternately referred to as Sound Preference)
3. Affrication/Deaffrication (or Sound Preference)
4. Cluster Reduction

Potential for increased intelligibility is another consideration. Although it is difficult to determine frequency of occurrence of the idiosyncratic processes in DE's case, the unusual and variable processes he used undoubtedly affected his intelligibility, giving another reason to target Spirantization. Grunwell (1985) suggests the inclusion of a contrastive analysis in addition to a process analysis. Considering the variability that interacts with the unusual processes in this case, a contrastive analysis might also be done. Intervention might then give priority to contrast development in early phases, with strengthening of the contrasts between stops, fricatives, and affricates in the system, and between coronals and other places of articulation.

Comparison of Goal-setting in Inventory and Phonological Process Approaches

Goals derived from a phonological process approach overlap with those from a developmental inventory approach, although the developmental approach may involve targeting the low frequency processes that affect the early segments such as /p/ and /t/, and with later attention to "later-acquired" elements such as liquids, affricates, and clusters. The inventory approach, furthermore, would not identify groups of segments that have common problems or lack of contrast between sound classes, but would consider /k/ separately from /g/, /s/ separately from /z/, with contrasts of stops and fricatives irrelevant. Independent of the framework used, there would be some overlap in intervention targets identified, partly because of limits on the set of possibilities. The convergence in targets suggests that the intervention plans will all lead to the same result: more adult-like speech. However, the aim is to arrive there in the shortest time possible. If a framework allows for a greater understanding of the system studied, more precise goal setting is possible. We noted that the inventory analyses fail to identify patterns. The process analysis identified some patterns, but had difficulty with the overlapping patterns and apparent variability.

In the next section, we show that a nonlinear analysis drawing on the concepts of Combinatorial Specification provides a more in-depth description and explanation of his phonological patterns and a more precise set of intervention targets.

Combinatorial Specification and DE's Phonological System

Although DE had some limitations on word structure his principal difficulties were related to features, and thus our nonlinear analyses focus on feature production: individual features, feature combinations, and feature sequences, in that order. As an introduction to the analysis, we first outline working procedures for the application of Combinatorial Specification to child data analysis.

Procedures in the Application of Combinatorial Specification to Child Data

Application of Combinatorial Specification to data analysis involves both independent (inventory) and relational (substitution) analyses. The segmental inventory and substitution analyses provide a basis for the feature analysis. The steps are:

1. *Determining inventories:* The segmental inventory and a guide such as Appendixes 1 and 2 provide a basis for determining the feature inventory. Presence and absence of individual features, feature combinations and feature sequences are noted.

2. *Identifying substitution patterns:* Substitution patterns are then identified for adult target features, combinations and sequences (as in a segmental substitution analysis).

3. *Default/nondefault determination:* At this point, Combinatorial Specification comes into play. The two main observations that lead to default determination are:

a. *Frequency:* Highly frequent features are often default features.

b. *Substitution status:* Default features often appear when the child does not produce a given segment with the target features for that segment.

For example, a child may produce stops for fricatives, suggesting that [–continuant] is the default value for [continuant]. Phones that are targets of assimilation often have default features. Stoel-Gammon and Stemberger (1994) note that coronals are often the target of assimilation patterns, supporting the concept of [Coronal] as the default place feature.

It is generally useful to start with the assumption that a child's defaults and nondefaults are identical to those of the adult target language. (See Appendixes 6–1 and 6–2.) Unmarked features in adult phonologies across languages are often default features. For example, voiced sonorants are more likely than voiceless sonorants. Thus, [+voice] is typically a redundant (default) feature for sonorants. Crosslinguistically, voiceless coronal stops are highly frequent, and hence the features [–continuant], [-voice] and [Coronal] are often default features and values.

Child-specific hypotheses are then considered when frequency and substitution patterns suggest such alternatives. (Combinatorial Specification allows for a child's defaults to be different from those of the adult, a fact of child phonology previously observed [Bernhardt, 1992; Bernhardt & Stoel-Gammon, 1996].)

4. *Feature combinations and defaults:* Types of feature combinations are then noted: default feature combinations, default and nondefault feature combinations, and nondefault feature combinations. If segmental complexity is relevant developmentally, we might expect combinations of defaults to appear developmentally earlier than combinations of nondefaults (Bernhardt & Stemberger, in press).

5. *Word position and sequence relevance:* Any differences in features and feature values across word positions are noted. These may arise from particular sensitivity to onset or coda constraints or from feature sequence constraints. As we mentioned earlier, Dinnsen (1996) suggests an extension of underspecification theory, Context-Sensitive Underspecification (suggesting specific onset or coda cooccurrence constraints). Sequences of features may show constraints. Ingram (1974) observed that labials are sometimes prohibited after other features, and Menn (1975), that velars are sometimes prohibited after other features.

If a child requires phonological intervention, selection of therapy targets involves further analysis procedures. We discuss such procedures after analyzing data from DE.

Analysis of DE's Data

Analysis of DE's data follows below, with Tables 6–3 through 6–8 showing feature inventories, substitutions, and combinations. The description of individual features follows the entire feature hierarchy from manner (Root) to Laryngeal to Place node features. The discussion of feature combinations and sequences is limited to those particular combinations and sequences that are most implicated in his phonological disorder (Tables 6–7 and 6–8). In the following sections, particularly significant difficulties are preceded by an asterisk and italicized.

Table 6–3. Features across word positions: Frequency chart.

Major Node	Feature	Word-initial	Medial Onset	Medial Coda	Word-final
Root	[–cons]	7	1		
	[+lateral]	1	0		2
	[+continuant]	41	8	2	15
	[–continuant]	14	15	1	20
	Branching [cont]	5			4
	[+nasal]	7	2	3	12
Laryngeal	**[+voice]**[a]	18	15	11	
	[–voice]	37	8	3	24
	[+spread glottis][b]	6			
Place	Labial	16	7		11
	Coronal [–ant]	3	0		0
	Coronal [–grvd]	0	0	0	0
	Coronal [+ant]	42	18	6	38
	Dorsal	0	0		0

Note: Numbers represent number of tokens in the sample for a given feature in a given word position.

Boldface: Features that are frequent in some word position in comparison with the opposite value for that feature in that word position.

[a]For obstruents only

[b]For voiceless stops only, where aspiration is required word initially

Features and feature combinations are described as established, developing or marginal. Minimum criterion level for establishment is 75% in terms of matches between the child forms and the adult targets. Marginal features match the adult target infrequently (15% or less). Features or feature values are considered frequent if prevalent both in absolute terms, and in comparison to contrasting features and feature values.

DE's Manner (Root) Features: Overview (see Tables 6–3 and 6–4)

All manner features were present across word positions, although with varying degrees of establishment:

1. [+nasal]: Established across word positions
2. [–consonantal]: Established for glides /w/ and /j/, developing for /r/
3. [+lateral]: Partially established word initially and finally

Table 6–4: Manner features: Matches, substitutions, and deletions for singleton stops, fricatives, affricates, and /l/.

Feature Target	Word-initial	Medial Onset	Medial Coda	Word-final
Fricatives: [+continuant]	✓ (13/18) ø (2) d, b: [–cont] ts: Branch [cont]	✓ (4/6) ø b: [–cont]	✓ (1/2) ø	✓ (13/14) ts: Branch [cont]
Stops: [–continuant]	✓ (7/19) s (8); z, f: [+cont] ts (2): Branch [cont]	✓ (12/15) ø (2) f: [+cont]	✓ (1/1)	✓ (16/17) ø
Affricates /tʃ/, /dʒ/: Branch [cont]	[s],[ʒ]: [+cont] [d]: [–cont]			✓ (2/3); z: [+cont]
/l/: [+lateral]	✓ (1/3) s, z: [+cons]-[–son]	ø (2) z: [+cons]-[–son]		✓ (2/5) ø (3)

Note: Assume 1 token where no number is given.
Bold: Feature established in some word position.
<u>Underlined:</u> Frequent substitution

---

*4. *[continuant]:* Partially established, with differences across word positions.

Because this feature was one of the key problems in his system (Affrication, Fricativization, and Stopping), we provide details in the next section.

DE's Production of the Feature [continuant]

As noted, [continuant] was variably realized across word positions. In word-final and medial onset positions, fricatives and stops matched the adult target in terms of manner. An exception occurred for *ice*, in which an affricate [ts] appeared for the fricative /s/.

(11)   truck   /trʌk/   [tʰʌt]
       vase   /veɪs/   [bes]
       makeup   /meɪk#ʌp/   [metəp]
       music   /mjuzɪk/   [musɪt]
       ice   /aɪs/   [aɪts]

Table 6–5: Laryngeal features: Matches, substitutions, and deletions for singleton consonants.

Feature Target	Word-initial	Medial Onset	Medial Coda	Word-final
[+voice][a]	✓ (12/12)	✓ (8/12) ø (2) s, t: [–voice]		✓ (9/10) ts: [–voice]
[–voice]	✓ (22/24) z (2): [+voice]	✓ (6/9) ø (2) z: [+voice]	✓ (2/3) ø	✓ (20/20)
[+spread glottis][b]	✓ (3/18) ø (2) (for /h/) s, f, ts: (12) [+cont][–vce] z: [+cont][+vce]			

Note: Assume 1 token where no number is given.
Bold: Established feature in at least some word position.
[a][+voice] for obstruents only. Note that /l/ and /j/ surfaces as [s] and [ts] respectively once each, i.e., [–voice].
[b][+spread glottis]: As a feature of the four /h/ targets, and for aspiration on 14 word-initial voiceless stops.

Table 6–6: Place features: Matches, substitutions, and deletions for singleton consonants.

Feature Target	Word-initial	Medial Onset	Medial Coda	Word-final
Labial	✓ (14/18) s (3), ts: Coronal	✓ (7/9) t, s: Coronal		✓ (9/10) z: Coronal
Coronal: [–anterior]	✓ (2/5) s (2), d: [–anterior]			ts (3), s (2): [+anterior]
Coronal: [–grooved]	z: [+grooved] d: [–cont]	d: [–cont]	s: [+grooved]	f: Labial
<u>**Coronal:**</u> <u>**[+anterior]**</u>	✓ (15/15)	✓ (11/12) ø		✓ (20/20)
Dorsal	s, (5), ts, z: Coronal	ø t, d: Coronal		ø t (6), d: Coronal

Note: Assume 1 token where no number is given; ✓ indicates feature match.
Bold: Established feature in at least some word position.
<u>Underlined:</u> Frequent substitution

Table 6–7: Selected feature combinations: Frequency chart.

Feature Combination	Segments Used	Word-initial	Medial Onset	Medial Coda	Word-final
[−cont]-[+voice]-[−nasal]	b, d	9	10		5
[−cont]-[−voice]-[−nasal]	p, t	4	4	1	13
[+cont][+voice][−son]	v, z, ʒ	7	5		7
[+cont]-[−voice]-[−son]	f, s, ʃ	32	4	1	8
Branch[cont]-[−voice]	ts	5			4
[−cont]-Coronal	t, d	6	9	1	12
[−cont]-Labial	p, b	7	5		6
Branch[cont]-Cor	ts	5			4
[+cont]-Coronal-[+anterior]	s, z	32			11
[+cont]-Labial	f, v	4			4
[+voice]-Coronal	n, j, l, r, d, z, ʒ	18	14		28
[−voice]-Coronal	t, s, ʃ, tʃ, ts	37	6		16
[+voice]-Labial	w, r, b, v, m	19	4		3
[−voice]-Labial	p, f	3	2		9

Note: Inventory includes singleton consonant productions for cluster targets.

Boldface: Denotes frequent combinations.

[a][−cont][−nasal]: Oral stops

Table 6–8: Feature combinations with [spread glottis]: Match proportions in word-initial position.[a]

Feature Combination in Target	Segments	Segment Match	Match [spread glottis]
[S:+voice]-[PR:–sp gl] [D:–cont] ---- [S: Lab], [D: Cor]	b, d	6/6[b]	6/6
[S:+voice][PR:–sp gl] [S:+cont] ---- [S: Labial]	v, w	3/4 /v/ > [b]	4/4[d]
[D:–voice]-[S:+cont] [PR:+sp gl] ---- [D: Labial]	f	3/6 /f/ > [s] (2), [ts]	6/6
[S:+voice]-[PR:–sp gl] [D:–cont]] ---- [S: Dorsal]	g	0/1 /g/ > [z]	1/1
[D:–voice] [D:–cont] ---- [S:+spread glottis], WI ---- [D: Coronal] ---- [S: Labial] ---- [S: Dorsal]	t p k	1/6 /t/✓, [s] (2), ts (2), z 0/2 /p/ > [s], [f] 0/6 /k/ > [s] (5), [ts]	5/6 (/t/ > [z]) 8/8
[D:–voice]-[S:+cont] [PR:+sp gl] ---- [D: Coronal]	s, ʃ, θ	3/4 /θ/ > [z]	3/4 ([+sp gl] > [–sp gl])
[S:+voice][PR:–sp gl]	z, ð, j	3/4	3/4

continued

Feature Combination in Target	Segments	Segment Match	Match [spread glottis]
[S:+cont] ---- [D: Coronal]	/ð/ > [d], /j/ > [ts]		([–sp gl] > [+sp gl])

Note: D = System default feature; PR = Phonetically redundant feature; S = Specified (nondefault) feature. Assume 1 token if no number is given.

[a]Because cluster targets involve word-shape constraints, these were not included. Note, however, word-initial /g/-clusters showed [s] substitutions 3/5 times, representing a change in [sp glottis].

[b]Proportions for *segments*, not [spread glottis]

[c]Feature changes listed under match proportion for segment

Thus, in these word positions, [continuant] appeared to be distinctive. Because there was no evidence to the contrary, we could assume adult default values, that is, [–continuant] as the default. Evidence supporting this hypothesis is the [ts] substitution for /s/. A [–continuant] feature was added in front of the target feature [+continuant], creating an affricate. (Substitutions generally have default values.)

In word-initial and medial coda positions, [continuant] values matched the adult target much less frequently: word-initial, 47/83 (57%) and medial coda, 3/5 (60%). Substitutions of [+continuant] or branching [continuant] for [–continuant] are apparent; that is, either a fricative or affricate ([ts]) for stop or affricate targets. As a substitution, [+continuant] appeared to be an example of a child "default" (the opposite of the default value in coda and medial onset positions). Dinnsen (1996) explains such cases with his theory of Context-Sensitive Underspecification. This may explain the difference in defaults between word positions. However, we will see below that difficulty with aspiration of voiceless word-initial stops ([+spread glottis]) may be more relevant here. This pattern in DE's speech occurred only for *voiceless word-initial* obstruents and the voiced velar (dorsal) stop /g/ (discussed in more detail in the section on feature combinations).

We noted that affricates were present in the sample, although not for all required targets. The presence of the affricate [ts] (as a substitution) indicates that branching structure of [continuant] was within DE's articulatory capacity, but was only partially established.

(12)   watch   /wɑtʃ/   [wats]   [ts]: Branch [continuant]
                                   default Coronal [+anterior]

| Joe | /dʒoʊ/ | [do] | [d]: default values of Coronal [+anterior], [continuant] |
| jump | /dʒʌmp/ | [ʒʌp] | [ʒ]: [+continuant], [−anterior]; ([−continuant] absent) |

DE's Laryngeal Features (see Tables 6–3 and 6–5):

1. [voice]: Established across word positions, although there is higher frequency of voiceless phones overall.

We can assume the adult default value of [−voice], because voiceless targets were produced with [−voice] and because the phone [s] was a frequent default segment, appearing in place of voiced targets (/z/ or /l/).

*2. [+spread glottis] (for /h/ and aspiration of word-initial voiceless stops): Marginal for voiceless stops, and developing for /h/.

hat	/hæt/	[æt]
hanger	/hæŋɚ/	[hɐ̃n]
truck	/trʌk/	[tʰʌt]
toothbrush	/tuθ#brʌʃ/	[tʰusrəʃ]
ten	/tɛn/	[zɛ̃n]
cup	/kʌp/	[sʌp]
page	/peɪdʒ/	[sets]

The segment [h] appeared 2/4 times, and aspirated stops, 4/21 times and only with [tʰ]. Word-initial /p/ was not present, and velars (dorsals) never occurred. In place of aspirated stops, coronal fricatives or affricates appeared. Thus the default for [spread glottis] was not [−spread glottis], as we might predict from adult English (which would give unaspirated stops); rather, the feature [+continuant] appeared. This is possibly the most interesting aspect of his substitution patterns. Because feature combinations and specification issues are implicated, we defer further discussion to the feature combinations section and the final discussion of Combinatorial Specification

DE's Place Features (see Tables 6–3 and 6–6)

*1. [Labial]: Developing across word positions.

The Place feature [Labial] is subject to cooccurrence and word position constraints, as we show in the section on feature combinations. Voiced labials were present in all positions, but voiceless labials consistently matched the adult target only in word-final position. The fricative /f/ was more often accurate than /p/ in non-final positions. Word-initial [p] never occurred. We return to this issue in the discussion of feature combinations.

book	/bʊk/	[bʊt]
rope	/roʊp/	[rop]
vase	/veɪs/	[bes]
watch	/wɑtʃ/	[wats]
fork	/fɔrk/	[sɔɪt]
four	/fɔr/	[foə]
paper	/peɪpɚ/	[fæfɚ]
page	/peɪdʒ/	[sets]
open	/oʊpən/	[otẽn]
zipper	/zɪpɚ/	[zɪpə]

2 [Dorsal]: Absent (no instances of /k/, /g/ or /ŋ/). Coronals [s] and [z] appear in their place word initially and coronals [t] and [d] in other positions.

coffee	/kɑfi/	[sɔsi]
couch	/kaʊtʃ/	[tsauts]
wrecker	/rɛkɚ/	[wɛdə]
gun	/gʌn/	[zʌn]
glasses	/glæsəz/	[sæsəz]

3. Coronal [−anterior]: Marginal. (Two matching tokens appear: [ʃ] for /ʃ/, and [ʒ] for the affricate /dʒ/.)
4. Coronal [−grooved]: Absent (no interdentals).
*5. *Coronal [+anterior]:* Established, and the major place substitution for labials, dorsals, and other features of [Coronal].

Thus, as is true of adult English, Coronal [+anterior] is the default place feature.

DE's Feature Combinations ("Paths")

Discussion of all feature combinations is not necessary to elucidate DE's major segmental difficulties. Hence, we focus on combinations of [continuant], [spread glottis], [voice], and Place, noted previously as particularly relevant. (See Tables 6–7 and 6–8.)

Voiceless word-initial stops were particularly problematic for DE, fricatives or affricates appearing often in their place. Fricatives also appeared for /g/ word initially, (either [s] or [z] as the examples given above for the feature [Dorsal] show). These are unusual substitutions in child phonology. We first suggested that the word-initial default for [continuant] might be [+continuant], in accordance with Context-Sensitive underspecification (Dinnsen, 1996). However, initial voiced stops /b/ and /d/ were accurately realized, and [b] and [d] also surfaced as substitutions for initial /v/ and /ð/, respectively.

(13) doll   /dɑl/   [dɑʌ]   [d]: [+voice]; [–continuant]
      this   /ðɪs/   [dɪs]   [d]: [+voice]; [–continuant]
      vase   /veɪs/   [bes]   [b]: [+voice]; [–continuant]

Hence, [–continuant] also appears to be the default. How can the system default for most voiced segments be [–continuant], and the system default for voiceless segments and /g/ be [+continuant]? This is not predicted by any underspecification theory. However, in the introduction, we discussed Default Underspecification as an extension of the theory of Combinatorial Specification. Some features are implied by other features (and are usually phonetically grounded). These are different from system defaults, which are particular to given languages or children.

Tables 6-7 and 6-8 contain the major clues to DE's unusual onset fricative substitutions. The major observation from those tables is that DE generally matched the laryngeal features of the target, independent of which other features surfaced. In the previous section, we noted that he had difficulty with aspiration of word-initial stops, and that we could therefore assume that the nondefault value of [+spread glottis] was only rarely produced. However, if we consider redundancies of the system, and all values of [spread glottis], we find that in fact he was faithful to the target in terms of all laryngeal features, including [spread glottis]. The features [spread glottis], [continuant], and [voice] have particular relationships when they combine because of **phonetic grounding**, resulting in the substitution patterns he showed. The following phonetic redundancies are relevant:

1. [+voice]–[–spread glottis]([continuant]): Voiced segments are redundantly [-spread glottis] in most languages. When the vocal folds are vibrating, they cannot be held in a spread position unless only one part of the folds is adducted, as with breathy voice. (Some languages, such as Hindi, do have breathy voiced obstruents, which are [+spread glottis].) The feature [continuant] can have either value in this combination. (Grounding condition II, a relative grounding condition.)

2. [–voice][spread glottis][–continuant]: Voiceless unaspirated stops are basically neutral with respect to the glottis. The state of the glottis does not allow vibration. As long as there is a chink, air can pass through. The glottis is [-spread glottis] in comparison with the spread position for aspirated stops. (Grounding condition II, a relative grounding condition.)

3. [–voice][+spread glottis][+continuant]: Voiceless fricatives are necessarily produced with [+spread glottis], for sufficient turbulence to be created. (Grounding condition I, an absolute condition).

DE adhered to the phonetic redundancies described here for these feature combinations, while apparently attempting to match the adult values for [spread glottis]. He matched voiced obstruents most of the time (except for /g/, which we discuss below). He matched voiceless fricatives most of the time. He matched voiceless stops in word-medial and word-final position most of the time.

DE had difficulty with the aspiration of word-initial stops and with /h/, both of which have [+spread glottis] features. He did manage to produce a few tokens of [tʰ] and /h/, but no other aspirated stops. The aspiration of word-initial stops, although present in English, is a marked phenomenon crosslinguistically. In trying to produce those marked aspirated targets, DE substituted voiceless fricatives or affricates, thus capitalizing on the phonetically grounded redundancy of [+continuant] and [+spread glottis].

Place features were sometimes vulnerable in his attempts to match laryngeal features. Very often, segments surfaced with the system default place, Coronal [+anterior]. The only aspirated stop was [tʰ], which was a combination of the default place feature and the marked nondefault laryngeal feature, [+spread glottis]. The most frequent word-initial substitution was [s], a combination of [–voice], [+continuant], [+spread glottis], and [Coronal]. Three of those features are defaults according to adult English ([–voice], [Coronal], and [+continuant] for [+spread glottis]). His attempt to match the [spread glottis] feature, and his difficulty with the combination of [–continuant] and [+spread glottis] thus made [s] a more likely word-initial substitution than the alveolar stops, which appeared as substitutions in other word positions. As we noted earlier, segmental complexity in terms of number of default and nondefault features can be relevant developmentally.

Particularly at risk were /p/ and the velars. Because /f/ is a voiceless fricative, it was favored by phonetic redundancies of [+spread glottis] and thus was developing. The /v/ was also developing, although, to maintain the [–spread glottis] feature, place, or manner was sometimes vulnerable. The realization of the nondefault [Labial] feature in combination with [+continuant] and [+spread glottis] was perhaps not a particularly difficult task, in comparison with the realization of a nondefault [Labial] or [Dorsal] feature with segments that did not have that [+continuant]-[+spread glottis] phonetic redundancy.

The production of /g/-clusters as [s] does not follow from the general redundancy patterns for [spread glottis]. One would expect a [d] or, at most, a voiced fricative, in keeping with his general patterns (given [d] for /ð/), and DE's attempt to match the laryngeal characteristics of the target. However, because [s] was a very frequent substitution, it could probably appear for /g/ also. If DE could not produce [Dorsal], all features of the target could be lost in the attempt to produce it. (Note that he also once used [s] for /l/, another voiced segment with a coronal place of articulation.) Bernhardt and Stemberger (in press) note that nonminimal repairs may occur in child phonology, with children deleting whole segments to avoid a feature or avoiding words altogether that have certain characteristics.

DE's Feature Sequences

One final comment can be made about words that had both voiceless labials and coronals as targets. In general, DE appeared to have an easier time producing voiceless labials *after* coronals than before them, or in context with other voiceless labials or nothing. (Lab = Labial; Cor = Coronal; ✓ = correct)

(14)	zipper	/zɪpɚ/	[zɪpə]	Cor . . Lab ✓
	paper	/peɪpɚ/	[fæfɚ]	Lab . . Lab ✓
BUT:	fork	/fɔrk/	[sɔɪt]	Lab . . Cor > Cor . . Cor
	open	/oupən/	[otɛ̃n]	Lab . . Cor > Cor . . Cor
	page	/peɪdʒ/	[sets]	Lab . . Cor > Cor . . Cor

Thus, in addition to the other feature constraints, a Labial-Coronal sequence constraint appears to have been present. This is unusual in phonological acquisition; Ingram (1974) observed that labials often appear in word-initial position only in early words. Nondefault features often appear to appear in prominent onset positions (Stemberger & Bernhardt, this volume).

Note that feature combinations with [Labial] and [+voice] were never subject to this sequence constraint , and that [f] was sometimes possible in this sequence.

(15)	basket	/bæskət/	[bæsɪt]	Lab-[+vce] . . Cor ✓
	rug	/rʌg/	[wʌd]	Lab-[+son] (=[+vce]) . . Cor ✓
	music	/mjuzɪk/	[musɪt]	Lab-[+son] (=[+vce]) . . Cor ✓
	football	/fʊt#bɑl/	[fʌtba]	Lab-[+cont] . .Cor . . Lab ✓
	flower	/flaʊɚ/	[flaʊ(w)ə]	Lab-[+cont] . . Cor . . (Lab?) ✓

The Labial-Coronal sequence constraint was thus not as powerful a constraint as other constraints in the system. Nevertheless, if there had been no sequence constraint, word-initial [f] would not have been in jeopardy in some targets, and the /p/ of *open* would possibly have been produced accurately. Note that the cases where [f] occurred before a coronal were also cases in which other labials followed in the word, with double linking of [Labial] possibly anchoring the [f] word onset. (See Stemberger and Bernhardt, Chapter 7, for a detailed description of the effects of sequence constraints.)

Summary

In summary, Combinatorial Specification, phonetic grounding, and Default Underspecification, an extension of Combinatorial Specification, are very relevant concepts for explaining DE's general patterns and much of the apparent variability noted in the process and inventory analysis. In his attempt to match laryngeal characteristics of a target, he sometimes failed to produce the target feature combinations. Manner features, although reasonably well established, were subject to phonetically grounded redundancies between [spread glottis], [voice], and [continuant] features. Place features other than default Coronal were weakly established and subject to individual feature constraints, feature combination constraints, and sequence constraints. In the next section, we consider how this analysis might influence intervention targets.

Intervention Goal Selection: Nonlinear Analysis and Combinatorial Specification

In this section, we present intervention goals that would arise from nonlinear analysis, in particular, from an application of Combinatorial Specification. Rationales for goal selection are provided. In general, this child might need to have easily attainable goals in the early phases of intervention because of a general feeling of low self-esteem about his speech. (Personality factors are considered alongside of phonological factors.) Throughout, we note whether the same or different goals were recommended by process and inventory analysis.

Segmental Goals for the First Intervention Period

Priorities for segmental level goals would be:

1. Aspiration of word-initial stops (and /h/)
2. Establishment of velars (dorsal)
3. Strengthening of [−anterior] (which can cooccur with [continuant] for branching structure of affricates) across word positions

Sequence of goals is addressed following further detail about each of them.

Aspiration of Word-initial Stops (and /H/. Targets are ([h]), [tʰ] > [pʰ], [kʰ]. The feature combination analysis showed the importance of this seemingly trivial (although marked) aspect of English phonology. Because he has already had some success producing [tʰ], [tʰ] would seem to be a reasonable first target. It might also be useful to target /h/ during this phase, showing him that a short [h] is the second part of the aspirated stop. Because [h] was already produced some of the time, this would presumably also be an attainable goal.

Whether [pʰ] or [kʰ] would be subsequent targets would depend on his ability to produce velars and the sequence of goals in the program. Typically, the aspiration phase of the velar is longer and noisier than the aspiration phase of the labial, and this length and noise may be facilitatory in intervention. However, aspirated [pʰ] has a stronger tactile sensation on the hand than aspirated [kʰ], and if tactile cues are important for a client, this might be the preferred next target. Within this intervention phase, it would be important to demonstrate the contrast between fricatives and aspirated stops. Note that this goal and the strategies to attain it would not necessarily be proposed after inventory and process analyses.

Establishment of Velars ([Dorsal]) Across Word Positions. The target is /k/ in word-final and word-medial onset positions, moving as quickly as possible to word-initial position for both /k/ and /g/.

Velars were missing, whereas most other features were at least partially established. Because /k/ is the most frequent of the velars, it has the potential to enhance intelligibility, once learned. Targeting /k/ in word-final position might be advisable, based on his more straightforward substitution of [t] word finally, and the finding that many children produce velars in codas before onsets (Stoel-Gammon, 1996). The other velars could serve as observation targets to evaluate generalization. Because the [s] substitution for velars detracts greatly from intelligibility, words with word-initial velars should be included as soon as possible in the treatment program. This goal and these strategies would also be selected after process and inventory analyses.

[*-anterior*] *Across Word Positions.* Targets are /ʃ/ (voiceless fricative) and /dʒ/ (voiced affricate).

Among the partially established features were:

a. Those for liquid specification ([+lateral]; Labial-Coronal)
b. Coronal marked features [–anterior] (alveopalatals) and [–grooved] (interdentals)

Of this group, the liquids already appeared in greater strength than [–anterior], and hence could remain baseline observation targets. Establishment of [–anterior] would circumscribe the Coronal [+anterior] default, and give an opportunity to reinforce the branching aspect of [continuant] by contrasting /ʃ/ and /dʒ/ as fricative/affricate and voiced/voiceless pairs. The other two alveopalatals could remain as observation targets to evaluate generalization. The interdentals are typically later acquisitions, and would not greatly enhance intelligibility in comparison with other targets. These goals were also selected following inventory and process analyses (deaffrication, depalatalization).

Syllable/Word Shape Goal Selection for the First Intervention Period

1. *Cluster production:* We would concur with the process and inventory analyses that word shapes with initial clusters would be a goal. Following our analysis, cluster targets would be selected that contain segments that are already well-established within his system, to circumvent powerful feature constraints. The following clusters would be possibilities:

a. /d/ and /b/ + sonorant (/bj/, /dw/ first, then possibly /bl/, /dr/, /br/)
b. /s/-clusters with sonorants /n/ or /m/

This set of clusters focuses on the two main cluster types (stop-approximant clusters, and /s/-clusters), and uses available segments, thus setting up the possibility for generalization across clusters. Clusters with the sonorant [w] were already in the system, suggesting that other obstruent-sonorant clusters such as /sn/, /sm/, /bj/, and /dw/ might be attainable. Because [fl] was present, /bl/ might be easily attainable, and /br/ and /dr/ might also be attainable, because /r/ was produced in several contexts. Other clusters, including word-final clusters could remain observation targets.

2. *Word position goals:* In terms of word position, it is clear that a major goal is improvement in overall match for word-initial position, both for singletons and clusters. This has already been addressed with segmental goal selection. However, there is another aspect to word position and segment production that has not been specifically addressed, namely the Labial-Coronal feature sequence constraint for voiceless labials.

Targets:

a. C_1 as /f/ with C_2 first as /t/, then /d/ < /z/ < /s/. Words of various lengths should probably be targeted, starting with the consonants appearing in two different CV syllables (e.g., *foo -ty*) articulated slowly and gradually increasing the speed of articulation, and moving to words with CVC syllables, breaking the syllable up as C-VC and CV-C (e.g., *f-it* versus *fi-t* > *muffet*). (It might be beneficial to introduce initial /v/ into this part of the program also, because voicing appeared to help circumvent the constraint on sequence, and DE must learn to produce /v/ in word-initial position.)

b. C_1 as /p/ with C_2 as /d/ < /z/ < /s/ in words of various lengths, as above.

DE was already experiencing some success with /f/. Once aspiration was possible, /p/ could follow.

This was not a goal identified from the process and inventory analyses.

Integration and Sequence of Segmental and Prosodic Level Goals Within the First Intervention Period

As stated, it would probably be important for DE to experience early success in the intervention program. Therefore, familiar, partially established targets would be goals of choice. A suggested order of goals for the first period is, then:

1. Segmental targets with some prior knowledge and some key role in his system:
   [+spread glottis] with [h] and [tʰ]
2. Word position targets with some prior knowledge:
   The Labial-Coronal sequence with /f/ (and perhaps /v/)
3. Segmental target with no prior knowledge:
   Velars ([Dorsal]) in non-word-initial position
4. Syllable-word shape target with some prior knowledge:
   Clusters with established segments: /bj/, /dw/, /sn/, /sm/, /bl/, /br/, /dr/
5. Segmental targets with some prior knowledge
   a. [+spread glottis] with [h] and [tʰ] as review, and word-initial [pʰ], [kʰ]
   b. [–anterior]: /ʃ/ and /dʒ/

Similarities between Nonlinear and Phonological Process/Inventory Analyses

Both nonlinear and process/inventory analyses capture aspects of the systematic patterns of the child's phonology, because they are both phonological analyses. Syllable structure development, segmental development, and idiosyncratic aspects of the system were addressed in the two methodologies. First period intervention targets determined by both methodologies included velars, fricatives/affricates, particularly alveopalatals, and possibly clusters. Segments chosen for those targets that matched were /k/ and alveopalatals.

Differences between Nonlinear and Phonological Process/Inventory Analyses

The nonlinear analysis, utilizing Combinatorial Specification, provided explanations for many of his apparently variable and idiosyncratic productions, particularly:

1. The unusual word-initial fricative substitutions: These were explained in terms of feature combination constraints and phonetically grounded redundancies for [spread glottis]. The fact that [s] appeared even for word-initial voiced segments /g/ and /l/ was attributable to underspecification theory also, in terms of frequency of use of default segments.
2. Inconsistencies with voiceless labial production: A labial-coronal sequence constraint was observed which further resulted in apparent variability in production of /f/ and /p/.

These analyses led to some different and more precise goals to address the main problems in the feature system.

CONCLUSION

Combinatorial Specification and phonetic grounding were useful concepts in the analysis of data from a child with a severe phonological disorder. Although the child's productions were variable, this variability was shown to arise primarily from feature combination constraints and redundancies for laryngeal features, particularly [spread glottis]. This analysis led to a more precise set of goals for intervention. Because the child's speech sample was collected many years ago, it is not possible to gather more to test our hypotheses with him. At some future point, we will have new data to evaluate the methodologies and theories. We hope that this overview has enhanced the readers' understanding of the benefits of application of certain aspects of grounded phonology, and will be assistive in future analysis and selection of intervention goals.

ACKNOWLEDGMENTS

The authors would like to acknowledge Dr. Joseph Paul Stemberger of the University of Minnesota for his insightful comments during preparation of this manuscript, and Michael Cam of the University of British Columbia for a very much appreciated computer speech analysis program.

REFERENCES

Archangeli, D. (1988). Aspects of underspecification theory. *Phonology Yearbook, 5,* 183–207.

Archangeli, D. & Pulleyblank, D. (1994). *Grounded phonology.* Cambridge, MA: MIT Press.

Avery, P., & Rice, K. (1989). Segment structure and coronal underspecification. *Phonology, 6,* 179–200.

Bernhardt, B. (1992). Developmental implications of nonlinear phonological theory. *Clinical Linguistics and Phonetics, 6,* 259–282.

Bernhardt, B., Doan, A., & Stoel-Gammon, C. (1995). Phonological and phonetic analysis of cleft palate speech. In K. Elenius & P. Branderud (Eds.), *Proceedings of the XIIIth International Congress of Phonetic Sciences,* Vol. 4 (pp. 108–115). Stockholm: KTH and Stockholm University Press.

Bernhardt, B., & Stemberger, J. P. (in press). Nonlinear phonology and child phonological development: A constraints-based analysis. San Diego: Academic Press.

Bernhardt, B., & Stoel-Gammon, C. (1994). Nonlinear phonology: Clinical application. *Journal of Speech and Hearing Research, 37,* 123–143.

Bernhardt, B., & Stoel-Gammon, C. (1996). Underspecification and markedness in normal and disordered phonological development. In C. Johnson & J. Gilbert (Eds.), *Children's language,* Vol. 9. (pp. 33–54). Hillsdale, NJ: Lawrence Erlbaum.

Chomsky, N., & Halle, M. (1968). *The sound pattern of English.* New York: Harper and Row.

Clements, G. (1987). Towards a substantive theory of feature specification. In *Proceedings of NELS 18* (pp. 79–93). Amherst: GLSA, University of Massachusetts.

Compton, A. (1970). Generative studies of children's phonological disorders. *Journal of Speech and Hearing Disorders, 35,* 315–339.

Dinnsen, D. (1996). Context-sensitive underspecification and the acquisition of phonemic contrasts. *Journal of Child Language, 23,* 57–79.

Dworkin, J. P. & Culatta, R.A. (1985). Oral structural and neuromuscular characteristics in children with normal and disordered articulation. *Journal of Speech and Hearing Disorders, 50,* 150–156.

Edwards, M. L., & Bernhardt, B. (1973). Phonological analyses of the speech of four children with language disorders. Unpublished manuscript. The Scottish Rite Institute for Childhood Aphasia, Stanford University, Palo Alto, CA.

Edwards M. L., Bernhardt, B., & Gierut, J. (1992). Three analyses for one phonologically disordered child. Different perspectives. ASHA *Convention Abstracts,* p. 146.

Grunwell, P. (1985). *Phonological assessment of child* speech. San Diego: College-Hill Press.

Hodson, B., & Paden, E. (1991). *Targeting intelligible speech: A phonological approach to remediation, Rev. ed.* (1983: San Diego: College-Hill Press) Austin, TX: Pro-Ed.

Howard, S. (1993) Articulatory constraints on a phonological system: A case study of cleft palate speech. *Clinical Linguistics and Phonetics, 7,* 299–319.

Ingram, D. (1974). Fronting in child phonology. *Journal of Child Language, 1,* 233–241.

Jakobson, R., Fant, G., & Halle, M. (1952). *Preliminaries to speech analysis: The distinctive features and their correlates.* (Technical Report 13, M.I.T. Acoustics Laboratory). Cambridge, MA: MIT Press.

Kiparsky, P. (1982). Lexical morphology and phonology. In I.-S. Yang (Ed.), *Linguistics in the morning calm* (pp. 3–91). Seoul: Hanshin.

Lombardi, L. (1991) *Laryngeal features and laryngeal neutralization.* Unpublished doctoral dissertation. Amherst: University of Massachusetts.

Macken, M. A., & Ferguson, C. A. (1983). Cognitive aspects of phonological development: Model, evidence, and issues. In K. Nelson (Ed.), *Children's language,* Vol. 4 (pp. 255–282). Hillsdale, NJ: Lawrence Erlbaum.

Maddieson, I. (1984). *Patterns of sound*. Cambridge, England: Cambridge University Press.

Masterson, J., & Pagan, F. (1993). *Interactive system for phonological analysis*. San Antonio: The Psychological Corporation.

McCarthy, J., & Prince, A. (1993). Prosodic morphology I: Constraint interaction and satisfaction. Unpublished manuscript. University of Massachusetts, Amherst.

Menn, L. (1975). Counter example to "fronting" as a universal of child phonology. *Journal of Child Language, 2,* 293–296.

Mester, A., & Itô, J. (1989) Feature predictability and underspecification: Palatal prosody in Japanese mimetics. *Language, 65,* 258–293.

Oller, D. K. (1973). Regularities in abnormal child phonology. *Journal of Speech and Hearing Disorders, 38,* 36–47.

Pulleyblank, D. (1986). Underspecification and low vowel harmony in Okpẹ. Studies in African Linguistics, 17, 119-153.

Rice, K. (1993) A reexamination of the feature [sonorant]: The status of "sonorant obstruents." *Language, 69,* 308–344.

Sagey, E. (1986). *The representation of features and relations in non-linear phonology*. Unpublished doctoral dissertation, Cambridge, MA: MIT.

Shriberg, L., & Kwiatkowski, J. (1982). Phonological disorders. III. A procedure for assessing severity of involvement. *Journal of Speech and Hearing Disorders, 47,* 256–270.

Stemberger, J., & Stoel-Gammon, C. (1991). The underspecification of coronal: Evidence from language acquisition and performance errors. In C. Paradis & J.-F. Prunet (Eds.), *The special status of coronals* (pp. 181–199). Dordrecht: Foris.

Steriade, D. (1987) Redundant values. *Chicago Linguistic Society, 23,* 339–362.

Stoel-Gammon, C. (1996). On the acquisition of velars in English. In B. Bernhardt, J. Gilbert, & D. Ingram (Eds.), *Proceedings of the UBC International Conference on Phonological Acquisition* (pp. 201–214). Somerville, MA: Cascadilla Press.

Stoel-Gammon, C., & Cooper, J. (1984). Patterns of early lexical and phonological development. *Journal of Child Language, 11,* 247–271.

Stoel-Gammon, C., & Dunn, C. (1985). *Normal and disordered phonology in children*. Austin, TX: Pro-Ed.

Stoel-Gammon, C. & Stemberger, J. P. (1994). Consonant harmony and underspecification in child speech. In M. Yavas (Ed.), *First and second language phonology* (pp. 63–80). San Diego: Singular Publishing Group.

Trubetzkoy, N. S. (1939). Grundzüge der phonologie. Travaux de Cercle Linguistique de Prague, 7. English translation (1969) by C.A.M. Baltaxe as *Principles of phonology*. Berkeley: University of California Press.

APPENDIX 6–1

Underlying Specifications for Adult English Consonants

Segment	Root (Manner)	Laryngeal	Place
/m/	[+nasal][a]		Labial
/n/	[+nasal]		c
[ŋ]	[+nasal]		Dorsal
/p/			Labial
/b/		[+voice]	Labial
/t/			
/d/		[+voice]	
/k/			Dorsal
/g/		[+voice]	Dorsal
/f/	[+continuant]		Labial
/v/	[+continuant]	[+voice]	Labial
/θ/	[+continuant]		Coronal: [–grooved]
/ð/	[+continuant]	[+voice]	Coronal: [–grooved]
/s/	[+continuant]		
/z/	[+continuant]	[+voice]	
/ʃ/	[+continuant]		Coronal: [–anterior]
/ʒ/	[+continuant]	[+voice]	Coronal: [–anterior]
/tʃ/	Branch [cont][b]		Coronal: [–anterior]
/dʒ/	Branch [cont]	[+voice]	Coronal: [–anterior]
/w/	[–consonantal]		Labial - Dorsal
/h/	[–consonantal]	[+spread glottis]	
/j/	[–consonantal]		Coronal [–anterior]-Dorsal
/l/	[+lateral]		
/r/	[–consonantal]		Labial-Coronal

Note: Only specified (nondefault) features are listed here.
[a][+consonantal] may be underlying, but is assumed to be redundant, given that consonants only appear in consonantal positions in the word.
[b][–continuant]-[+continuant] for affricates.
[c]Coronal [+anterior] is assumed to be the default for place, hence is unspecified.

APPENDIX 6–2

Full Specifications for Adult English Consonants[a]

Segment	Root (Manner)	Laryngeal	Place
/m/	[+consonantal][+nasal]		Labial
/n/	[+consonantal][+nasal]		Coronal: [+anterior]
[ŋ]	[+consonantal][+nasal]		Dorsal
/p/[b]	[+cons][–continuant]	[–voice] ([+spread glottis])[b]	Labial
/b/	[+cons][–continuant]	[+voice]	Labial
/t/[b]	[+cons][–continuant]	[–voice] ([+spread glottis])[b]	Coronal: [+anterior]
/d/	[+cons][–continuant]	[+voice]	Coronal: [+anterior]
/k/[b]	[+cons][–continuant]	[–voice] ([+spread glottis])[b]	Dorsal
/g/	[+cons][–continuant]	[+voice]	Dorsal
/f/	[+cons][+continuant]	[–voice]	Labial
/v/	[+cons][+continuant]	[+voice]	Labial
/θ/	[+cons][+continuant]	[–voice]	Coronal: [–grooved] [+distributed]
/ð/	[+cons][+continuant]	[+voice]	Coronal: [–grooved] [+distributed]
/s/	[+cons][+continuant]	[–voice]	Coronal: [+anterior]
/z/	[+cons][+continuant]	[+voice]	Coronal: [+anterior]
/ʃ/	[+cons][+continuant]	[–voice]	Coronal: [–anterior]
/ʒ/	[+cons][+continuant]	[+voice]	Coronal: [–anterior]
/tʃ/	[+cons]Branch [cont][b]	[–voice]	Coronal: [–anterior]
/dʒ/	[+cons]Branch[cont]	[+voice]	Coronal: [–anterior]
/w/	[–consonantal]		Labial [+round]-Dorsal
/h/	[–consonantal]	[+spread glottis]	
/j/	[–consonantal]		Coronal [–ant]-Dorsal
/l/	[+cons][+lateral]		Coronal: [+anterior]
/r/	[–consonantal]		Labial-Coronal
/ʔ/	[–consonantal]	[+constricted glottis]	

[a]Only English redundancies are included. Crosslinguistic phonetic redundancies are not included here. See Appendix 6–3 for some examples.
[b]In word-initial position, voiceless stops are aspirated, i.e., have a feature [+spread glottis].
[c]Coronal [+anterior] is assumed to be the default for place, hence is unspecified.

APPENDIX 6–3

Some Examples of Phonetic Redundancies

Feature	Root	Laryngeal	Place
[+sonorant][a]		[+voice] OR [+spread glottis][a]	
[+consonantal]			PLACE[b]
[−sonorant]	[+consonantal] [−nasal] [−lateral]		PLACE[b]
[−consonantal][c]	[+sonorant] [+continuant] [−lateral]	[+voice] OR [+spread glottis]	
[+lateral][d]	[+sonorant] [+continuant] [−nasal]	[+voice]	PLACE[b]
[+nasal]	[+sonorant] [−continuant] [−lateral]	[+voice]	PLACE[b]
[+continuant]	[−nasal]		
[−continuant]	[+consonantal] [−lateral]		PLACE[b]
Branch [cont]	[+consonantal] [−sonorant] [−nasal]		PLACE[b]
[+voice]		[−spread glottis]	PLACE[b]
[−voice]	[+consonantal] [−sonorant] [−lateral] [−nasal]		
[+spread glottis]	[+continuant][e]	[−voice]	
Labial	[−lateral]		
[+anterior]	[+consonantal]		
[−anterior]			Coronal [+grooved]
[+grooved]			Coronal
Dorsal			[+back][f]

continued

Note: When a feature is not mentioned in columns 1–3, alternate values of that feature may apply to the feature in Column 1, i.e., there is no necessary phonetic redundancy.

[a]The feature [+sonorant] is not necessarily [-consonantal], because nasals are consonants. Furthermore, it is not necessarily [+continuant], because nasals are noncontinuant (continuants being produced with oral airflow.) It is not necessarily [+voice] because /h/ is voiceless, and vowels, liquids, and nasals can be voiceless in some languages. In such cases, the sonorant is necessarily [+spread glottis]. However, a voiceless sonorant may still pattern as a sonorant phonologically, and thus be classified as [+sonorant] even though not spontaneously voiced (see Lombardi, 1991; Mester and Ito, 1989; Rice, 1993.)

[b]Noncontinuants have oral place features, and liquids and nonglottal glides have oral place features.

[c]The segment /h/ is [−consonantal] and [+sonorant] (Chomsky & Halle, 1968) but is not voiced. See Footnote [a] argumentation.

[d]Laterals may act as glides ([−consonantal]) or consonants ([+consonantal]). This is true of /r/ also, although it is more glide-like in English in many contexts than /l/.

[e]The portion of an aspirated stop that is [+spread glottis] can be considered [+continuant].

[f]Vowels also are considered to have Dorsal place, and may have different redundant features.

CHAPTER

7

Optimality Theory

JOSEPH PAUL STEMBERGER
BARBARA HANDFORD BERNHARDT

In this chapter, we explore the implications of **Optimality Theory** (OT) for speech-language pathology. The major sources for the theory are Prince and Smolensky (1993) and McCarthy and Prince (1993), and, for acquisition, Bernhardt and Stemberger (in press). But at the time of writing, the most accessible readings in OT for the speech-language pathologist are found in Bernhardt, Gilbert, and Ingram (1996). The first part of the chapter outlines major aspects of OT, and the second part discusses application of this theory to phonological intervention, giving general guidelines and a specific case example.

In its approach to the analysis of phonological patterns, OT focuses on two important aspects of any phonological system: the patterns that are impossible and the patterns that are possible. It is distinguished from most other approaches to phonology in the extreme role that is assigned to **constraints**:

Constraint is a limit on what constitutes a possible pronunciation of a word. Optimality theory uses only two mechanisms for determining the pronunciation of a word: the underlying representation of the morpheme or word (often referred to as the **input**), and constraints. OT does not account for differences between input and output form in terms of processes or rules, but in terms of constraints. We will make clear exactly how constraints and rules are different, and why OT leads to a different sort of analysis than process-based approaches.

Although OT has been developed only recently, it is related to a number of previous theories. Within approaches to child phonology, it combines a relational approach and an independent approach. It requires us to examine a child's pronunciations of words as reflecting the child's independent phonological system, while also focusing us on the ways that the child's system (and hence the child's pronunciation) matches or differs from the adult's system (and hence from the adult's pronunciations). It is also related to a number of earlier approaches to phonology. In the 1970s, Stampe (1973) suggested that all human beings have the same set of natural processes, and OT similarly assumes that all human beings have the same set of constraints. Hooper (1976) proposed that phonological systems should not have both processes and constraints; but she argued that processes can be used to express constraints on phonological forms. In terms of recent theories, most linguists working within an OT framework presuppose nonlinear phonology (see the chapters by Bernhardt & Stoel-Gammon, Dinnsen, and Ingram, this volume). In addition, OT has borrowed a number of assumptions from connectionist theory as laid down by psychologists (e.g. Rumelhart & McClelland, 1986), leading to a perspective that is different from other linguistic theories in many ways.

THE THEORY

Basic Issues in Optimality Theory (OT)

In this section, we review the role of constraints in OT, showing why constraints have a different focus than processes. We also introduce the concept that some constraints are more important than others, and that the less important constraints can sometimes be ignored (**violated**).

One important viewpoint in the analysis of child phonology is the relational approach. A comparison is made between the adult and child pronunciation and similarities and differences are noted. In the process approach to child phonology (e.g., Ingram, 1976; Hodson, 1986), the focus is on the *differences* between the child and adult forms, and on the aspects of the adult pronunciation that the child does not have. For example, if the word *big* (adult /bɪg/) is pronounced [bɪ], we talk of Final Consonant Deletion. Although this is useful, it ignores some very important information: the matches between the adult and child forms. In the pronunciation [bɪ], the child accurately produces the initial consonant and the vowel; the process approach accounts for this fact obliquely (if no processes are noted that would affect an initial consonant or a vowel), but does not draw our attention to it. OT draws attention not just to differences between child and adult pronunciations, but also to similarities. As a result, the practitioner of OT gives the child credit for the child's partial mastery of the adult system, drawing attention to points of strength that can be used by the clinician to build up more adult-like pronunciations.

OT further provides a framework for the analysis of *adult* languages that makes the child's phonology seem less different than the process analysis often suggests. Because adults have mastered the phonology of their native language, we tend to forget that there are many things that adults cannot do in their language. All languages have constraints that limit an adult's performance. In OT, the child has some constraints that are not important for adult speakers of the language; but other constraints may hold true for both children and adults. Many generalizations can be made about pronunciations of words by any speaker of any language (whether an adult or the youngest child). For adult English, some of these generalizations are absolute:

- No word may end in /tp/ (as in */rɪtp/), though /pt/ is possible.
- No word may start with */tl/ or */dl/, but /pl/, /bl/, /tr/, and /dr/ are possible.
- No word may start with */mr/ or */nr/, though /br/ and /fr/ are possible.
- No word begins with [ŋ] (as in *[ŋɪp]),
- No word contains the voiced fricatives *[ɣ] (velar) or *[β] (bilabial).

None of these constraints hold true of every adult language. Spanish has the fricatives [ɣ] and [β]. Vietnamese can begin a word with [ŋ]. Slovenian can begin a word with [mr]. Russian can begin words with /tl/ and /dl/. Seri can end words with /tp/ (Moser & Moser, 1965). But all of these constraints are important for adult speakers of English. New words (such as the names of commercial products like laundry detergent) always abide by these constraints. Speakers of English learning foreign languages initially have difficulty with words that violate these constraints.

Other generalizations about English are concerned with how frequent certain patterns are:

- Very few words start with two fricatives (as in *sphere*).
- Relatively few words begin with an unstressed syllable (as in *banana*).

Speakers of English are not aware of having difficulty with these low-frequency phonological patterns, but their low frequency may make them more difficult for adults to process.

Many theories of phonology require us to account for such generalizations (via constraints) and to account for the fact that different languages show different limits on possible words. This is not necessarily true in a process approach, which focuses on other types of phonological patterns. If a pattern is observable only because it never occurs in the underlying representation of any word, the process approach does not necessarily have to address the pattern.

Additional generalizations about phonological patterns involve **alternations** in the language, in which a morpheme shows two or more pronunciations in different (phonological) contexts. For example, there is a [t] at the end of the word *sit* when it appears by itself, but the /t/ is pronounced as a tap [ ] between vowels (in words and phrases such as *sitting* [sɪN] and *sit on* [sɪ ʌn]), and as a glottal stop [ʔ] before a syllabic /n/ (in the colloquial pronunciation *sittin'* [sɪʔən]). In some theories, such alternations are captured via **processes**: a "rule" that changes the /t/ into the tap [ ] or the glottal stop [ʔ] in particular phonological environments. A process approach *must* contain processes to account for alternations, but generally does not contain processes to account for patterns that do not involve alternations.

In OT, there are no processes, even for alternations. All phonological generalizations are made using constraints. Constraints and not processes cause alternations. Some constraints are absolute limits on the pronunciation of words: the constraint can never be violated. For example, no English word can start with */dl/. However, other constraints do not hold absolutely. There are exceptions in which the constraint is violated. For example, the constraint in English that the first syllable of the word must be stressed is violated in a relatively small number of words (including *machine* and *banana*). Such violable constraints express patterns that are frequent, but not true of all words in a language. In fact, *every word violates some of the constraints of the language*. The concept of violable constraints is a major distinguishing characteristic of OT.

The speaker's goal is to pronounce a word using the **optimal** ("best") pronunciation of that word. To do so, the speaker must determine which constraints are most important. Some constraints are very important and may never be violated. Other constraints are less important and can be violated. Some constraints are very weak and can be freely violated. The *optimal* pronunciation of the word does not violate the very important constraints; it violates the least important constraints. OT provides us with a detailed set of constraints on pronunciations, along with a **ranking** of the constraints from most important (high-ranked) to least important (low-ranked). The pronunciation of each word is shaped by the constraints that it violates and by the relative importance of those constraints. Because different languages (and different children) show the effects of different constraints, it is clear that constraints differ in their ranking (importance) in different languages (and in different children).

Some constraints prevent particular phonological elements (such as particular features) from being in pronunciations. For example:

(1) **Not([+lateral])**: lateral consonants ([l]) are not allowed.

For a language such as English, such a constraint potentially causes problems, because /l/ appears in English words such as *little* [lɪdɫ]. Thus, this constraint against laterals is in conflict with a second constraint:

(2) **Survived([+lateral])**: If the word has a lateral consonant in it, that lateral consonant must be pronounced.

Whether or not the speaker produces [l] depends on which of these two constraints is ranked higher; the symbol "»" denotes that the constraint on the higher line (or sometimes on the left) is ranked higher than the constraint on the lower line (or sometimes on the right):

(3) **Survived([+lateral])**
     »
     Not([+lateral])

The more important constraint is **Survived**, which requires the speaker to pronounce any lateral consonants that are present in the underlying representation of a word; as a result, [l] is pronounced. The lower-ranked constraint **Not([+lateral])** is violated—one could say that the lower-ranked constraint is "ignored." As adult speakers of English can pronounce [l], this is the ranking that they have. However, suppose that the ranking were in the opposite order:

(4) **Not([+lateral])**
      »
      Survived([+lateral])

In this case, it is more important that there be no laterals in the pronunciation. If any words contain /l/ in the underlying representation, the /l/ must not be pronounced. This could be accomplished by omitting the segment entirely, or by producing something else in its place:

(5) *light* /laɪt/ → [aɪ] or [waɪ] or [jaɪ] or [daɪ] or . . .

Although no (normal) adult speaker of English has this ranking, young children often do. All the variant pronunciations listed here have been reported for different children. The substitution that appears in a given child's speech for the impossible /l/ is determined by other constraints.

This example illustrates the basic workings of OT. There are often two constraints in conflict, each requiring a different pronunciation. The higher-ranked constraint is the one that determines the actual pronunciation. In essence, the ranking constitutes a theory of *ease of articulation*. However, OT differs from previous ease-of-articulation theories: What is difficult for one person (or language) need not be difficult for another (because the constraints are ranked differently). Furthermore, learning ("practice") can result in something difficult becoming easy (as in phonological development or sound change).

Some Basic Constraints

In OT, there are two types of rankable constraints. Both make reference to the **output**: the actual pronunciation. One type also makes reference to the **input**: the underlying (or lexical) representation of a word (or morpheme). Although both are often called "output" constraints, because they refer to what is allowable in the output, they have different functions, and it helps to think of them as two different (often opposing) forces. The two types of constraints are:

Faithfulness: The output must correspond to the input with respect to <something>.

Output: The output may not contain <something> **or** must contain <something>.

Faithfulness constraints are necessary, because they ensure a lexical component to the pronunciation. Output constraints refer purely to what is possible in the output, without reference to the input. If given free rein, the output constraints would lead to every word in the language being produced with the same optimal output (presumably [baba] or [titi]) (McCarthy & Prince, 1994). Faithfulness constraints prevent that and force the speaker to use pronunciations that reflect each individual morpheme. For some children (very young or very disordered), faithfulness may be ranked low enough so that almost every word is pronounced the same.

The faithfulness constraints help ensure that lexical information in the underlying representation is present in the surface pronunciation. We deal with only one faithfulness constraint in this chapter, which relates to the elements and association lines that are present in the underlying representation. We highlight our constraint names (from Bernhardt & Stemberger, in press) with a pencil icon "✐" and note other names for the given constraints (used by different researchers adopting an OT framework) with a scissors icon "✂." We have attempted to make our constraint names transparent and will use them throughout this chapter (but the reader will encounter other names elsewhere in the literature and thus we also note them).

In the descriptions that follow, we give definitions of constraints, describe violations of the particular constraints, give other names for the same constraint, and indicate what the general basis ("grounding") for the constraint might be. (See below for a more in-depth discussion of grounding, and Bernhardt and Stoel-Gammon, this volume.)

✐ **Survived**: An element in the underlying representation must be present in the surface pronunciation.
Violation: A deleted element (i.e., absent from the output).
Other names: ✂MAX,✂Corr(i,o),✂Containment.
Grounding: Communicative/functional (maintain lexical information).

Survived is a family of constraints; there is one for every feature or node in the feature geometry (see Ingram, Chatper 2): **Survived([+voiced]), Survived(Labial), Survived(Root)**, and so on. **Survived(Link)** prevents the deletion of underlying association lines. Elements (such as features) must remain linked up in the surface pronunciation (i.e., occur at the same point in time in the word) in the same way that they are in the underlying representation; **Survived(Link)** prevents features from migrating from their original place in the word into some other segment. Cole and Kisseberth (1994) have argued that **Survived** is ranked higher in "strong prosodic positions" (onsets, stressed syllables, word-initial position) than in "weak prosodic positions" (codas, unstressed syllables, word-final position); faithfulness is thus more likely to be violated in weak positions than in strong positions.

Most approaches to OT also assume a faithfulness constraint that prevents the insertion of elements and association lines that are not present in the underlying form. This has been called ✂RecFeat, ✂LexFeat, ✂DEP, ✂Corr(o,i), and (for some functions) ✂Fill. However, we are not convinced that a faithfulness constraint is needed to prevent epenthesis. Epenthesis and other insertions are prevented by other constraints that are needed independently.

In opposition to faithfulness constraints are output constraints that impose their own shape on surface pronunciations. We regard the "negative" (**Not, NotCooccurring**, etc.) constraints as the most important core set of constraints. The grounding for most of these constraints is cognitive, lying in information processing. All actions require the use of limited cognitive resources, and some actions require more resources than others. A high-ranked negative constraint implies that an element requires many resources; a low-ranked negative constraint means that few resources are required. It should be emphasized that *all* elements require *some* resources; thus, there are negative constraints against *all elements*.

The most important negative constraint is **Not**:

☞   **Not**:   An element must not appear in the output.
        Violation: The element is present in the output.
        Other names: ✂*Struc; ✂NoCoda; ✂*(Element); ✂LexFeat; ✂LexLink.

One of the functions of this constraint is faithfulness. **Not** prevents elements from appearing in the output, and therefore also prevents the *insertion* (or epenthesis) of elements in the output. An element is possible in the output only if there is a higher-ranked constraint that requires it to be there. If the only relevant higher-ranked constraint is **Survived**, then underlying elements are possible in the output, but insertion is not possible. Insertion occurs when some other constraint that requires an element is ranked higher than **Not**, as we address below.

Smolensky (1993) has shown that the relative ranking of the members of the **Not** constraint family determines the phonological **defaults** of the language (see Bernhardt & Stoel-Gammon, this volume, for discussion of defaults). Consider, for example, the following ranking:

(6)   **Not(Dorsal)** » **Survived(Dorsal)** » **Not(Labial)** » **Not (Coronal)**

The ranking of the two constraints on the left prevents the feature [Dorsal] from appearing in the pronunciation of consonants. Underlying /k/, /g/, and /ŋ/ cannot be pronounced as velars. However, if a consonant is still pronounced with a place feature, that place feature must be [Labial] or [Coronal]. Given the ranking of the two constraints on the right, the underlying velars will surface as coronals: Velar fronting, with /k/→[t], /g/→[d], and /ŋ/→[n]. They cannot surface as labials (/k/→[p]), because **Not(Labial)** is more important (ranked higher) than **Not(Coronal)**. If a consonant must have some place of articulation, it is optimally [Coronal]. Given this ranking, when the [Dorsal] feature of the velars cannot survive, the optimal place feature [Coronal] is inserted. Note that labials can still be pronounced as labials (/p/→[p]), as long as **Survived(Labial)** is more important than **Not(Labial)**; all underlying labial consonants must preserve their underlying features and surface as labials. Bernhardt and Stemberger (in press) note that, if we assume underspecification, it is possible to leave underlyingly coronal consonants like /t/ and /n/ unspecified for [Coronal] in the underlying representation; as **Not(Coronal)** is the lowest-ranked **Not** constraint for place of articulation, [Coronal] will be filled in automatically, with /t/ surfacing predictably as alveolar [t].

A second negative constraint prevents two elements from occurring in the same segment, or in general at the same point in time:

✑   **NotCooccurring(A,B)**: A and B may not cooccur at the same point in time.
      Violation: A and B cooccur at the same point in time.
      Other names: ✄PathCond; ✄*Clash; ✄CodaCond; ✄*M; ✄*P.

This constraint plays a very large role in the grounded phonology of Archangeli and Pulleyblank (1994) (see Bernhardt & Stoel-Gammon, this volume). Smolensky (1993) has proposed that the relative ranking of the different members of the **NotCooccurring** family are correlated with the relative rankings of the members of the **Not** constraint family. If **Not(A)** is ranked higher than **Not(B)**, then **NotCooccurring(A,C)** is ranked higher than **NotCooccurring(B,C)**. This follows from resource demands: if A generally requires more resources than B, it will require more resources when it combines with other elements.

We also make use of a positive version of this constraint family:

✏ **Cooccurring(A→B)**: If A is present, then B must also be present at
          the same point in time.
    Violation: A occurs without B at the same point in time.

A typical instance of this constraint is **Cooccurring ([+sonorant] →
[+voiced])**, which requires sonorant consonants and vowels to be voiced
(Itô, Mester, & Padgett., 1995). Bernhardt and Stemberger (in press) also
makes extensive use of the following type of constraint:

   (7)   **Cooccurring(Rime→<vowel-features>)**

Such constraints require that any segment in the rime of a syllable,
whether a vowel or a consonant, must have vowel features such as
[+sonorant], [-consonantal], [Dorsal], [+continuant], and so on. They can
lead to features such as [Dorsal] and [+continuant] being allowed in
coda consonants but not in onset consonants; see elaboration following.
    A third negative constraint prohibits sequences of elements:

✏ **NoSequence(A. . .B)**: Given two segments, the sequence A followed
          by B is impossible.
    Violation: The sequence A followed by is present.
    Other names: ✄ClustCond; ✄Generalized OCP; *(AB).

Most of the time this constraint family involves place or manner features, for example, **NoSequence(Coronal. . .Labial)**, or **NoSequence
([-nasal]. . .[+nasal])**.
    A related constraint prevents a sequence of two identical elements.
In theory, this could be a special type of **NoSequence** constraint, but
repetition seems to cause special problems for cognition in general
(Norman, 1981), so we regard it as a separate constraint:
✏ **NotTwice**: An element may not appear twice if the two tokens are
          adjacent.
    Violation: Two adjacent tokens of an element.
    Other names: ✄OCP; ✄*Echo.

NotTwice can rule out a sequence of identical segments (e.g., */pp/), or
a sequence of identical features (*[Labial][Labial], as in *[pm]).
    Another negative constraint prevents an element from being pro-
duced for an extended period of time:

✏ **SinglyLinked**: An element can link upwards to only a single higher
          element.

> **Violation**: A doubly-linked element.

This prevents double linkage. Among other things, this constraint is active in languages in which long vowels and/or long consonants are impossible. In English, **SinglyLinked(C-Root)** is ranked high, so long consonants (*[atːi]) are not possible; but **SinglyLinked(V-Root)** is ranked low, so that long vowels are possible (*boot* [buːt]).

The last negative constraint that we will present here prevents a node in the feature geometry (see Ingram, this volume), from containing more than one element on lower tiers:

☞ **NotComplex**: An element may link downwards to only a single lower element.
> **Violation**: Consonant clusters within an onset or coda or diphthongs (complex nuclei).
> **Other names**: ✄*Complex.

This plays an especially strong role in limiting the complexity of prosodic structure.

The constraints that we have addressed so far are grounded in communicative and cognitive functions. Some constraints may have phonetic grounding. However, phonetic grounding more commonly has its expression not in the *presence* of constraints, but rather in the *ranking* of constraints. Archangeli & Pulleyblank (1994) presuppose that constraints such as **NotCooccurring([–ATR],[+high])** (segments cannot simultaneously have a high tongue body *and* a non-advanced tongue root) is present because of phonetic grounding. We assume that this constraint is present for cognitive reasons, reflecting the general problem of producing multiple elements at the same time; but it is ranked higher than **NotCooccurring([+ATR],[+high])** for phonetic reasons that reflect physical constraints on the tongue.

One phonetically grounded constraint is that all representations must be complete enough to be programmed phonetically. For example, if a Place node is present, then it must link downwards to *some* articulator feature. This has been called ☞**LinkedDownwards** and ✄Fill.

Working with Constraints

Phonological patterns arise from different rankings of basic simple constraints. The challenge of phonological description is in determining the *relevant* constraints for a given pattern and the relative importance (ranking) of those constraints. Consider the following ranking of constraints:

(7)   **NoSequence(Coronal. . .Labial)**
      »
      Survived(Labial)
      »
      Not(Labial)

Generally, [Labial] is accurately produced (**Survived(Labial)** » **Not(Labial)**). However, [Labial] may not follow a coronal consonant, and may be deleted after coronals; deleting [Labial] after [Coronal] avoids the violation of the high-ranked **NoSequence** constraint, at the cost of violating **Survived(Labial)**. A sequence as in *top* /tɑp/ loses the labial: [tʰɑt] (Stemberger, 1993).

This example illustrates one of the major characteristics of OT. What could be stated as a process (change labials into coronals after coronals) is unpacked into a set of constraints. A process is made up of a change and an environment (where the change occurs). The change part of a process corresponds to the violation of a faithfulness constraint in OT. The environment corresponds to one or more output constraints. By unpacking the process into its parts, we can more clearly see that different processes are related to each other. For example, a child might change /l/ into [j] in onsets *(light* [jaɪt]), [ʊ] in codas *(fall* [faʊ]), and [u] when syllabic *(apple* [ʔapu]). All of these patterns are motivated by **Not([+lateral])** and its interaction with other constraints. We predict that it will be common for two or more such processes to affect the same element, but in different ways. Further, we predict that there might be multiple ways to avoid a sequence that violates a constraint, depending on the environment. In a process approach, the similarities between different changes are obscured. In OT, they are highlighted.

Within OT analyses, the interest lies in determining how the different constraints interact. To a large degree, it is a matter of determining which faithfulness constraints tend to be obeyed, and which tend to be violated. For example, suppose a child has no [l], reflecting the high ranking of the **Not([+lateral])** constraint. Consider the possible alternative outputs for the word *light* /laɪt/:

(8)   /l/ is deleted: [aɪt]
              violates: **Survived(Segment)**
      /l/ → [j]:   [jaɪt]
              violates: **Survived([+consonantal]), Not([−consonantal]),
                            Not([−anterior])**

/1/ → [w]:   [waɪt]
    violates: **Survived([+consonantal]), Not([–consonantal]),**
                Not(Labial)
/1/ → [z]:   [zaɪt]
    violates: **Survived([+sonorant])**
/1/ → [d]:   [daɪt]
    violates: **Survived([+sonorant]), Survived([+continuant])**

Each of these possible alternative pronunciations avoids violating the constraint against the feature [+lateral], but each does so at a cost. There are other features that must also change if [+lateral] is eliminated. But whether another feature can be changed depends on the ranking of the faithfulness constraints for that feature. The relative importance of those other constraints determines which other features survive or are changed, and thus directly determines how the word is pronounced.

Summary

We have introduced the concept of constraints and discussed how they are related to (but also differ from) processes. In review, constraints can be ranked to reflect their relative importance, that is, low-ranked constraints can be violated. It is the interaction of different constraints that determines the pronunciation of a word. In this section, we have presented a subset of important phonological constraints which are useful in describing acquisition data. Because the constraints of OT unpack processes into several parts, we can achieve a more integrated picture of a phonological system and explicitly see the relationships between different processes—often seeing the *reason* that a particular process is present in a language or a child's system. In the next section we discuss the application of OT to phonological disorders, both generally and for a specific case example.

APPLICATION TO PHONOLOGICAL DISORDERS

Background

In the 1970s, the field of speech-language pathology adopted analytic methodologies from linguistics. Phonological process analysis became the most commonly used methodology for the description of a child's speech sound (phonological) disorders (e.g., Edwards & Bernhardt, 1973;

Hodson, 1986; Ingram, 1981). In addition to developmental norms, factors such as the relative frequency of phonological processes, intelligibility, rule/process ordering, and potential for generalization were considered relevant during goal selection. In recent years, nonlinear phonological theory has provided a basis for new developments in phonological intervention (Bernhardt, 1992a, 1992b; Bernhardt & Stoel-Gammon, 1994; Bernhardt & Stoel-Gammon, this volume). Such applications of nonlinear theories predate Optimality Theory (OT), but do assume constraints in addition to or in place of rules/processes. Development is viewed as a positive progression: Over time, children learn to overcome a number of prosodic and segmental constraints. Developmental norms, frequency of error patterns, intelligibility, and potential for generalization remain key factors in goal selection.

OT, as a formalized theory of constraints, provides an opportunity for development of more refined constraint-based applications of nonlinear phonological theory. Constraint-based theory provides a deeper understanding of a child's phonological system and predicts certain learning phenomena and certain rules-of-thumb for clinical intervention. In addition, some of the specific constraints discussed in the introduction bring new insights for resolving clinical problems.

General Advantages of OT for Intervention

Getting to the Root of the Problem

By trying to understand *why* certain phonological patterns exist, we may be able to find faster ways of facilitating change in those patterns. For example, when a child produces [t] for /k/, **Not(Dorsal)** is high-ranked, prohibiting velars. But there are many ways a child could avoid producing velars: from replacement of [Dorsal] with [Coronal] (Velar Fronting) to the more drastic replacement with a (placeless) glottal stop or deletion of the entire segment. Which alternative solution results depends on the ranking of other constraints in the system, as we have discussed in the introduction. Examining the speech of many children, it will often be found that the same process results from very different constraint interactions, because other aspects of the children's phonological systems are different.

Arriving at a general constraint ranking for a phonological system is a time-consuming process. However, knowing the relationships of the various constraints can help in intervention planning, suggesting potential hazards and benefits of inclusion or exclusion of certain targets and contexts. For example, when a child finally develops fricatives in codas, it may reflect a high ranking for the constraint **Cooccurring(Rime→ [+continuant])**. This suggests that it may be relatively easy to acquire other consonants with vowel features in codas, such as velars or sonorants. Segmental context of an entire word is often also relevant. If a child produces alveolar stops not only for velars but for many other segments, the best words to use for training velars should probably not contain alveolars elsewhere in the word, either as targets or potential substitutions. Such remedial rules-of-thumb have been part of the clinician's practical knowledge for some time (see Kent, 1982; Grunwell, 1985; Bernhardt, 1992a). But with constraint-based theory and particularly the OT version of it, we now have a better way of examining relationships among phenomena and a theoretical basis for explaining why some of the clinical rules-of-thumb are effective.

Understanding Changes During Intervention

The goal of intervention is to accelerate phonological development in the direction of normalcy. Whatever the theoretical basis for an intervention program, some changes generally occur. At times there appears to be more regression than progress, as children begin to overgeneralize new structures or segments. For example, a child learning velars may, for a time, produce velars for coronals (e.g., *top* /tɑp/ [kʰɑp]), even though coronals previously replaced velars. Rule/process theory does not predict such regressions. The new rule/process (backing) can be described (as the opposite of the previous process of fronting), but there is nothing in process theory itself that explains the overgeneralization. OT, however, provides a theoretical basis for such changes. Generally, in OT, a change in output reflects a change in constraint rankings. If a child learns to produce velars, **Not(Dorsal)** becomes lower-ranked than faithfulness constraints for [Dorsal] (**Survived(Dorsal)**). But it may also accidentally become lower-ranked than **Not(Coronal)**, making [Dorsal] the new default place feature in the child's system, and resulting in regressive overgeneralizations for alveolar consonants:

(9) *Child's Ranking*   *Adult Ranking*
     Survived(Dorsal)   **Survived(Dorsal)**
     »   »
     Not(Coronal)   versus   **Not(Dorsal)**
     »   »
     Not(Dorsal)   **Not(Coronal)**

The OT framework, with its adjustable constraint rankings, has a formal mechanism to account for such learning phenomena.

Utility of Specific Constraints

Certain constraints appear to be particularly important in development. One of the key competitions in OT is between something and nothing. During speech, humans are compelled to be faithful to their linguistic input, to communicate; thus, **Survived** constraints should be high-ranked. On the other hand, it is easier to communicate with a minimum of effort; thus, the **Not** constraints compete for top ranking with the **Survived** constraints. For children, particularly those with processing, motoric, or anatomical limitations, **Not** constraints tend to outrank faithfulness constraints. Development entails a gradual lowering in ranking for **Not** constraints, with a concomitant higher ranking for faithfulness constraints. Contemplating the process of change in terms of this competition may lead a clinician to purposefully seek activities that emphasize the communicative function of utterances, such as contrast activities. This does not suggest anything new for therapy, but it does support and explain why a communicatively functional approach may be efficacious for some children. It also may explain why some children are slow to progress: Such children may not have the energy, ability, or interest to exert the effort required to overcome high-ranked **Not** constraints.

Specific constraint types that have proven particularly useful in explaining phonological patterns are the cooccurrence constraints (also a key part of Archangeli & Pulleyblank's, 1994, theory of combinatorial specification). Bernhardt and Stoel-Gammon (this volume) describe the utility of that theory for explaining apparently variable patterns in the speech of one child with a phonological disorder. Previous phonological theories had little to say about within-segment context (features). OT incorporates this strength.

Rime cooccurrence constraints are useful in explaining positional differences for segment realization. Features that are more vowel-like may appear in the rime, and features that are more consonantal may appear in onsets. As noted above, if a child shows some evidence of rime cooccurrence constraints, this may be something that intervention can exploit.

Sequence constraints have been previously identified in child phonology (Ingram, 1974; Menn, 1975; Stoel-Gammon, 1983). Stemberger (in press) argues that such constraints can underlie a number of phonological patterns, such as metathesis or assimilation. In the next section of this chapter, we present a case study of a child who has extensive consonant harmony: assimilation of consonant features across vowels, as in [kʰɪk] for *tick* /tɪk/. We provide an analysis showing how high-ranked **NoSequence** and **Not** constraints could underlie this process and discuss the intervention strategies that were effective in reducing the impact of those constraints. We turn now to that case study, and consider additional possible applications of OT to phonological intervention in the conclusion of this chapter.

Case Study: Harry (From Ages 4;5 to 4;8)

Although a number of developmental phonologists have begun to analyze child phonological data in terms of OT (see Bernhardt et al., 1996), application to phonological intervention has been minimal. For the case study we have chosen to present, a constraint-based framework was applied to determine goals and strategies. Major competing constraints were identified, although detailed rankings were not worked out prior to intervention. Before proceeding to the case discussion, we review key points about constraints typically relevant to consonant harmony, the child's major process.

Overview of Constraint Interactions Resulting in Consonant Harmony

Stemberger (in press) suggests that consonant harmony has two major motivations: **NoSequence** constraints and constraints related to feature (under)specification.

a. **NoSequence** constraints usually result in leftward harmony. Consider **NoSequence(Coronal. . .Labial)**, which underlies the impossibility of words like */rɪtp/ in adult English. Although it simply says that the two place features may not appear in that order, it often leads to surface patterns in which the second feature (Labial) is affected. This is because the second feature is in a weak prosodic position (non-word-initial position), where faithfulness constraints are less important than in strong positions (such as word-initial position; Stemberger, 1992; Cole & Kisseberth, 1994). Developmentally, initial consonants appear earlier than final consonants. As a child learns to produce final consonants, there can still be limitations on which final consonants are possible. Default features often fare best in codas. Constraints against such features are ranked lowest, and the default features are consequently easiest. (Sometimes, however, rime cooccurrence constraints can promote vowel-like features, which are typically nondefault features in consonants.) When nondefault features become possible in final position, they may only be possible if pronounced in (linked to) more than one prosodic position. Double linking to an onset places the feature in a strong prosodic position, making it more likely to survive. But spreading a non-default feature such as [Labial] to an earlier consonant position entails the loss of whatever place feature originally appeared in that position. Typically, default Coronal place is more often a target of consonant harmony than other features: A nondefault feature may only be able to link up to a Place node in which there are no other nondefault features.

How does leftward (anticipatory) consonant harmony look in terms of constraints? The following constraint table shows constraint interactions for the production of *tip* as [pʰp̄]. Constraint tables (see Table 7–1) are a useful graphic device for showing constraint interactions. Alternative candidate pronunciations for the input (upper left cell) are listed in the top row. Relevant constraints are listed in the first column, with the higher-ranked constraints higher in the list. An asterisk indicates that a constraint is violated in that alternative pronunciation; an exclamation point after the asterisk (plus a special border) reflect a fatal violation (the violation that makes that alternative pronunciation less than optimal). The candidate pronunciation that is optimal given this constraint ranking is enclosed in a special border. Cells in which violations do not matter are lightly shaded.

The sequence and faithfulness constraints for the nondefault features are high-ranked (reflected in the fatal violations for [tʰp̄] and [tʰɪ]). The child wants to produce the nondefault feature but *cannot* do so if the preceding feature is a default feature. The low ranking of **SinglyLinked(Nondefault)** means that there is no strong constraint against the double linking of features. Both [tʰɪ] and [pʰp̄] violate that constraint, but that is permissible because the constraint is low-ranked. The ranking of **Not(Default)** is higher than **SinglyLinked(Nondefault)**; otherwise, [tʰp̄] would be preferred to [pʰp̄]. Leftward harmony is often due to sequence constraints.

Table 7–1. Constraint table example.

/tɪp/	[tʰɪp]	[tʰɪt]	[pʰɪp]
NoSequence(Default. . .Nondefault)	*!		
Survived(Nondefault)		*!	
Not(Default)	*	*	
SinglyLinked(Nondefault)			*

Also, underspecification may also underlie harmony, especially if it is both rightward (perseveratory) and leftward. In such cases, nondefault features typically appear in place of default features, whether they occur before or after the default feature in the target; the particular order of features is irrelevant, unlike in Table 7–1. Critical constraints concern the features themselves and particularly the relationships between nondefault and default features. A consonant with default features is underlyingly underspecified for those features and must obtain a feature in some fashion. One way is to produce a segment with default features, but another way is to borrow a nondefault feature that is present in a nearby segment; either way, some feature is present in the surface pronunciation. To prevent harmony, the following ranking is needed:

(10) **SinglyLinked(Nondefault)**
»
Not(Default)

Given this ranking, it is easier to insert a default feature (violating the lower-ranked constraint) than to spread an existing feature from another segment (violating the higher-ranked constraint). But if the constraints are in the opposite order, harmony results:

(11) **Survived(Nondefault)**
Not(Default)
»
SinglyLinked(Nondefault)

This ranking can lead to both rightwards and leftwards harmony (Table 7–2). Now that we have presented sufficient background, we turn to Harry's case study.

Data and Analysis, Harry

Harry's data were collected and transcribed by his speech-language pathologist. The sample size is small for each data point (49 words of the Hodson, 1986, word list) but not atypical of samples collected in clinical practice. Although we cannot answer all analysis questions adequately with such a sample, it serves as a good test of the application of linguistic theories under the severe time constraints of clinical practice. Bernhardt analyzed the data following each probe, and, together with the clinician, designed the intervention plans. Harry progressed well during the program and entered kindergarten with intelligible speech.

Table 7–2. Constraint tables for consonant harmony.

/pɪt/	[pɪt]	[tɪt]	[pɪp]
Survived(Nondefault)		*!	
Not(Default)	*!	*	
SinglyLinked		*	*

/tɪp/	[tɪp]	[tɪt]	[pɪp]
Survived(Nondefault)		*!	
Not(Default)	*!	*	
SinglyLinked		*	*

This case study contains a detailed analysis of his assessment data, the initial intervention plan with goals and strategies, and a summary of the follow-up probes and subsequent intervention plan. We first address syllable and word structure, then feature and segmental development, and finally, the pervasive consonant harmony process. Key goals and strategies suggested by the data are noted at the end of each analysis subsection, with a summary of the intervention plan given at the end of the analysis.

Syllable Structure, Harry's Phonology

All the words in the sample were produced with the correct number of syllables (up to four syllables). Syllable structure was limited, however. Clusters were absent. Codas were also subject to deletion (absent in 6/22 CVC words); nasals were the only sound class impervious to the **Not(Coda)** constraint. This suggested high ranking for a rime cooccurrence constraint, **Cooccurring(Rime,[+nasal])**.

(12)   smoke   /smoʊk/   [mo]
         slide   /slaɪd/   [tæ]
         mask   /m{sk/   [m{]

mouth	/mʌʊθ/	[mɔʊ]
nose	/noʊz/	[no]
star	/stɑr/	[dɑ]
leaf	/lif/	[ti]
horse	/hɔrs/	[toʊə]

The syllable structure analysis led to these suggested intervention goals and strategies:

Goals: Codas, clusters

Strategy: Rime cooccurrence constraints might be operating, suggesting introduction of vowel-like features in coda consonants.

Consonant Features, Harry's Phonology

Harry's pronunciations included labial and coronal stops and nasals, a few approximants (occasional medial [w] and [l], and glottal stop), and one word-final affricate, [ts].

(13)	mouth	/mʌʊθ/	[mɔʊ]	Labial, [+nasal]
	nose	/noʊz/	[no]	Coronal, [+nasal]
	basket	/bæskət/	[bæpeɪp]	Labial, [−continuant]
	truck	/trʌk/	[tʌt]	Coronal, [−continuant]
	yellow	/jɛloʊ/	[ʔʌlo]	[+c.g.], [−cons], [+lateral], Coronal
	jump rope	/dʒʌmp roʊp/	[mʌʔwop]	Labial, [+nasal], [+c.g.], [−cons]

Velars, fricatives, and the glides [r], [j] and [h] were not produced. Coronal stops replaced fricatives (including labiodentals), dorsals, glides (including /h/), and liquids (unless the consonants were subject to labial or nasal harmony). Note the loss of [Labial] in the labiodental fricatives.

(14)	shoe	/ʃuː/	[tu]
	three	/θriː/	[ti]
	yoyo	/joʊjoʊ/	[dodo]
	fork	/fɔrk/	[doʊt]
	vase	/vɑz/	[dɑ]
	leaf	/lif/	[ti]
	horse	/hɔrs/	[toʊə]
	truck	/trʌk/	[tʌt]
	snake	/sneɪk/	[neɪt]

Nondefault features were:

Root:	[+nasal]	[m], [n]
	[+lateral]	[l]
	[−consonantal]	[w], [ʔ]
Place:	[Labial]	[m], [b], [p], [w]

Default features were:

Root:	[−continuant]	[p], [b], [t],[d], [m], [n], [ʔ]
Laryngeal:	[+constricted glottis]	[ʔ]
Place:	[Coronal]	[t], [d], [n], [l]

Feature combinations were:

Labial, [−continuant], [+voice]	[b]
Labial, [−continuant], [−voice]	[p]
Labial, [+nasal] ([−continuant])	[m]
Labial-Dorsal, [−consonant],	[w]
Coronal, [−continuant], [+voice]	[d]
Coronal, [−continuant], [−voice]	[t]
Coronal, [+nasal]	[n]
Coronal, [+lateral]	[l]

Missing features and feature combinations were:

[+continuant], [−sonorant]	*fricatives
[+spread glottis]	*[h]
[−consonantal], Labial-Coronal	*[r]
[−consonantal], Coronal	*[j]
Dorsal	*velars

Voicing matched the target only some of the time.

The feature system was minimally established for a child of this age. High-ranked faithfulness constraints for nondefault features were:

(15)   **Survived(Labial)**
        Survived([+nasal])
        (Survived([+lateral])): marginal, since [1] surfaced only occasionally

High-ranked **Not** constraints prohibiting nondefault features and combinations were:

Not(Dorsal)

Not([+spread glottis])

NotCooccurring([+continuant],[−sonorant])

NotCooccurring(Labial,Coronal)

Low-ranked constraints promoting defaults and harmony were:

Not([-continuant])

Not(Coronal)

SinglyLinked(Labial)

The feature analysis led to these suggested intervention goals and strategies:

Goals: [Dorsal], [+continuant,−sonorant], and [+lateral] greatest needs.

Strategy: [Dorsal] and [+continuant] might be best elicited in coda first, because of Rime Cooccurrence constraints that favor vowel-like features in rimes.

Summary of Repairs/Processes for Word Structure and Features

Many repairs were **minimal**: involving just the feature that caused the constraint violation. This included velar fronting and stopping (of fricatives and liquids). The prohibited features failed to link up, and default features (Coronal, or [−continuant]) were inserted in their place.

A number of repairs went beyond the level of the prohibited feature, however: pervasive default insertion, segment deletion, consonant harmony, and reduplication. Coronal stops not only replaced dorsals and sibilants, but also [h] (which does not have a place feature) and labiodental fricatives. Thus, coronal stops acted as pervasive defaults. Segment deletion was another **nonminimal** repair, always affecting consonants in clusters and sometimes affecting consonants in codas. Labial and nasal consonant harmony were also highly frequent. All of these "processes" result in major simplification and homonymy across the system. We noted in the introduction to this case study that consonant harmony may be a response to feature underspecification. The general lack of feature development in Harry's system suggests that underspecification may be a strong motivation of harmony. In the next section, we discuss this further.

Consonant Harmony

Harry had both labial and nasal harmony. Labial harmony was generally bidirectional, but was only leftwards in monosyllables when it cooccurred with nasal harmony (compare *mouth* and *gum*). Nasal harmony was only leftwards, except when nasal and labial harmony cooccurred (as in the word *music box* [mumitʌ]). Harmony did not always affect onsets in stressed syllables, where the default insertion of [Coronal] occurred instead (see *television, music box, crayons*).

Leftwards Nasal Harmony:

(16)	queen	/kwin/	[nin]
	string	/strN/	[nin]
	crayons	/kreɪjʌn+z/	[teꞑʌn]
	television	/tɛlɘvɪʒɘn/	[tɛnɘnꞑɘn]
	Santa Claus	/s{ntɘklʌz/	[n{nɘtʌ]
BUT:	mask	/m{sk/	[m{]
	nose	/noʊz/	[no]

Leftwards Labial Harmony:

soap	/soʊp/	[bop]
ice cubes	/(ʔ)aɪʃ kjubz/	[paꝑub]
zipper	/zɪp /	[bꝑʊ]
jump rope	/dʒʌmp roʊp/	[mʌʔwop]
cowboy hat	/kaʊbɑ h{t/	[pʌbɑd{ʔ]

Rightwards Labial Harmony:

page	/peɪdʒ/	[peꞗ]
boat	/boʊt/	[bop]
basket	/b{sk@t/	[b{peꝑ]

Labial and Nasal Harmony together (resembling reduplication):

> *Leftwards:*
> gum   /gʌm/   [mʌm]
> thumb   /θʌm/   [mʌm]

> *Rightwards:*
> music box /mjuzɪk#bɑks/ [mumitɑ]

Leftwards Nasal Harmony plus rightwards Labial Harmony:

>   plane   /pleɪn/   [meɪm]
>   spoon   /spun/   [mum]
> BUT: mouth   /mʌʊθ/   [mɔʊ]

As shown above, *faithfulness* constraints for the nondefault features [Labial] and [+Nasal] were high-ranked in comparison to the **Not** constraints for those features. **SinglyLinked** was low-ranked for those features, allowing double linking.

(17) **Survived(Labial)**
       Survived([+nasal])
       »
       Not([+nasal])
       Not(Labial)
       SinglyLinked(Labial)
       SinglyLinked([+nasal])

To account for the range of patterns, additional rankings are needed. We first address the cases in which harmony did not apply to all syllables of a multisyllabic word, and then proceed to discuss the directionality issue, which is more relevant in terms of intervention strategies.

HARMONY IMMUNITY FOR SOME STRESSED SYLLABLES.   In words of more than one syllable, onsets of some stressed syllables unexpectedly showed no harmony effects. Coronal stops (either as matches or substitutions) surfaced in onsets in such cases, with the default features [Coronal] and [−continuant].

(18)	crayons	/kreɪænz/	[teɪ̃nʌn]
	television	/'tɛlɘvɪæn/	['tɛ̃nɘ̃nɪ̃nɘ̃n]
	Santa Claus	/'sɪntɘklʌz/	['nɪ̃nɘ̃tʌ]
	music box	/'mjuzɪk(ˌbʌks)/	['mumi(ˌtʌ)]
	cowboy hat	/'kaʊbɔɪ(hɪt)/	['pʌbɔɪ(dˀ)]
BUT:	ice cubes	/aɪskjubz/	[paˌpub]

Word length was irrelevant to the pattern. Apparently, **SinglyLinked** was higher ranked for strong prosodic positions like onsets than for weak positions like codas. [Labial] could violate this for onsets only when [Labial] was underlying in onset (and thus reinforced by the presence of an underlying link).

However, *ice cubes* was exceptional to this pattern. The syllable with primary stress *did not resist* harmony. This vowel-initial word had no underlying features in the onset (assuming that glottal stops are inserted word-initially). Therefore, [Labial] was not blocked from spreading. In order for [Labial] to be realized phonetically, default features [-continuant] and [-voice] were inserted (to create [p]). The data suggest that underlying feature structure can block spreading in the stressed syllable onset, even by an empty Place node (as for the coronal stop in *television*, and *crayons*), or a [+consonantal] Root feature (/h/ of *hat*). (Although /h/ is often considered a glide, the substitution of [d] for /h/ some of the time suggests that /h/ was [+consonantal] in Harry's system). High-ranking of **Cooccurring([+consonantal]→C-Place)** leads to insertion of C-Place and [Coronal]. (For further discussion of such implicational redundancies, see Bernhardt and Stoel-Gammon, Appendix 6-3, this volume.)

This part of the analysis led to the following *suggested intervention goals and strategies*. The harmonizing process was not absolute, and thus could probably be broken down further through intervention that: (1) took syllable prominence and foot structure into account, and (2) gave special attention to vowel-initial words.

DIRECTIONALITY. The directionality issues are also intriguing, and relate to both types of motivation for harmony: sequence constraints and underspecification. Why was nasal harmony generally limited to a leftwards pattern (except when [Labial] also spread)?

(19)	string	/strɪN/	[nin]	leftwards
BUT:	snake	/sneɪk/	[neɪt]	NO HARMONY
	spoon	/spun/	[mum]	leftwards for [+nasal]
				rightwards for [Labial]
BUT:	mask	/mɪsk/	[mɪ]	NO HARMONY

The strong constraint on the direction of nasal harmony in mono-syllables suggests a sequence constraint for that feature. Nasals could *precede* other nasals, glottal stops or no consonant, but nasals could not *follow* nonnasals: **NoSequence([–nasal]. . .[+nasal]).** Default-nondefault sequences are often subject to sequence constraints, as we noted above. The leftwards direction of the repair is consistent with this type of sequence constraint. This constraint is also active for the leftwards vowel nasalization process in adult English ([bĩn] for /bɪn/ but not *[nɔ̃b] for /nɔb/).

(20) Labial harmony, in contrast, was bidirectional:

plane	/pleɪn/	[meɪm]	rightwards
boat	/boʊp/	[bop]	rightwards
page	/peɪdʒ/	[peɪb]	rightwards
soap	/soʊp/	[bop]	leftwards
ice cubes	/aɪs kjubz/	[paɪpub]	leftwards

Feature (under)specification probably motivated labial harmony much of the time, leading to bidirectionality. Labial harmony occurred when there was a default place feature in the target (*boat, plane*) or when other nondefault features in the target (whether place or manner features) could not be produced. In other words, [Labial] was generally realized wherever it could appear, given the stressed syllable constraints noted above, and the following restriction.

In the monosyllable examples *mask* and *mouth*, coda deletion occurred rather than rightwards labial harmony. Rightwards labial har-mony was possible, as we have noted (see [peɪb] for *page*). However, nasal harmony was not rightwards in monosyllables. Perhaps [Labial] could not copy or spread independently of [+nasal] when these features cooccurred. Such a restriction may suggest copying/reduplication of segments (spreading of Root plus features) rather than spreading or copying of autonomous lower-level features. However, note that most examples of double linking respected the voicing of the target (*page, ice cubes*). Since exact Root (segment) copies would have identical voicing feature, the data therefore suggest that features are copying or spread-ing, with some kind of additional constraint on independent spreading of the place feature when cooccurring with [+nasal].

These intervention goals and strategies were suggested:

Goal: Harmony reduction
Strategies:
a. Nasal harmony could possibly be reduced through an approach that targeted alternating sequences of nasals and nonnasals. The lack of

harmony in nasal-nonnasal sequences might help to inhibit harmony in the subsequence nonnasal-nasal sequence (e.g., ma-da-ma-da-ma-dam > *madam*).

b. Focusing on development of segments with nondefault features other than [Labial] might reduce the amount of labial harmony, given the hypothesis that pervasive harmony derived from the lack of nondefault features.

c. In early stages of therapy, the interaction of the two harmonizing features should be kept in mind (see strategies below for Labial-Coronal sequences).

Summary of Relevant Constraints

Throughout the analysis, we identified several major constraints. Ranking of these various constraints resulted in the various patterns observed. Generally, the following rankings were pertinent. (Different rankings of some of these occurred for specific segments or structures some of the time.)

(20) **SinglyLinked(Onset$_{-Strong}$):** prohibits harmony in onsets of some stressed syllables

NotComplex(Onset/Coda): prohibits clusters
»
Survived(Labial): allows labials
Survived([+nasal]): allows nasals
Survived([+voice]): allows voiced stops
Cooccurring(Rime→[+nasal]): facilitates nasal in codas
Not(Dorsal): prohibits velars
Not([+continuant]): prohibits fricatives
Not([+lateral]): prohibits /l/
»
Not(Coda): prohibits codas
» *(unstable ranking)*
Survived(Dorsal): allows velars
Survived([+cont]): allows fricatives
Survived([+lateral]): allows /l/
SinglyLinked(Labial): allows labial harmony
SinglyLinked([+nasal]): allows nasal harmony
Not(Coronal): default place
Not([−continuant]): default manner
Not([−voice]): default voice

Intervention Plan: Treatment Block I

At the time of intervention, goals and strategies were identified, although not expressed in terms of constraint rankings. According to OT, constraint rankings need to change for outputs to change developmentally. Here we identify what rerankings were needed, as an adjunct to goal and strategy description.

The following were given priority for the first treatment phase:

a. Reduction of labial harmony:
   Constraint reranking: higher ranking of **SinglyLinked(Labial)**
b. Nondefault feature development (tied in with the reduction of labial harmony):
   Constraint reranking: higher ranking of **Survived** for nondefault features other than [Labial] and [+nasal]
c. Coda enhancement (tied in with the first two goals):
   Constraint re-ranking: lower ranking of **Not(Coda)**
   Constraint exploitation: Cooccurring(Rime→<vowel-features>)

These goals were addressed in the following ways.

Labial harmony reduction was addressed by (a) targeting sequences of Labial-Coronal consonants in CVCV and CVC, and (b) by targeting nondefault features.

(a) Labial-Coronal sequences were targeted rather than Coronal-Labial sequences, because progressive harmony is less common than regressive, and Labial-Coronal sequences are generally less restricted in English (as noted in the introduction to this chapter). Two limitations on labial harmony were considered when constructing stimuli sets:

(i) The resistance of onsets in stressed syllables to harmony

(ii) The interaction of nasal and labial harmony in terms of the rightward-restricted directionality of labial harmony for /m/.

Thus, CVCV words with equal (strong) stress were used for the introduction of Labial-Coronal sequences, and /m/ was used some of the time in the first syllable. Stimuli such as *Bah Dee* or *Me Dee* were repeated in gradually faster alternations until words such as *Body (meaty)* resulted. Once he could pronounce the Labial-Coronal sequence in CVCV, the final vowel was dropped (*Bod, meat*).

(b) Nondefault feature establishment

(i) [+continuant]: /h/ in onset, /s/ in coda

Fricatives are a major sound class. Because /h/ is placeless, the feature [+continuant] can be the main focus of production for that segment.

The /s/ is frequent and has default place and voice features. Because [Labial] did not survive in fricatives (/f/→[t]), coronal fricatives were therefore more optimal first targets than /f/ or /v/. Harry had a tendency towards high-ranked rime cooccurrence constraints (nasal codas were strong), and thus the coda might be an optimal first choice for the establishment of fricatives with an oral place of articulation. By targeting /h/ in onset and /s/ in coda, a wide scope for the feature [+continuant] was provided: cooccurrence with place versus with laryngeal features, and with both onsets and codas.

(ii) [+lateral]: Liquids are another major sound class. Harry produced /l/ once in the initial probe, and hence /l/ was considered an achievable target.

(iii) Coda enhancement: Codas were not directly targeted. However, by targeting /s/ in coda, and Labial-Coronal sequences in CVC words, the coda constituent itself could be strengthened.

Results of Block 1 Intervention

Harry made notable gains in the first treatment block (approximately 10 weeks).

1. *Harmony*: There was a reduction in frequency of progressive labial harmony. He became capable of producing Labial-Coronal sequences in disyllables and monosyllables. Coronal-Labial sequences remained problematic.

A **NoSequence(Coronal. . .Labial)** constraint became visible, as a cause of regressive labial harmony. [Labial] was sufficiently strong in onsets at this point, but not yet in codas unless doubly linked to onset.

Nasal harmony was not directly addressed, nor did it decrease in frequency.

2. *Nondefault features*: Fricatives and affricates appeared ([+continuant]), particularly fricatives and affricates. A [ts] appeared for coda sibilants, /ts/, and /ks/ (all in conversation) and for word-initial /f/ (in therapy situations). The [h] appeared some of the time in conversation. The /l/ was also produced in therapy contexts.

In terms of constraints, **Survived([+continuant])** became higher-ranked, but usually in conjunction with [−continuant] (in affricates). **Cooccurring(Rime,[+continuant])** was usefully exploited in intervention. Interestingly, [f] was produced only in onset, even though the sibilants were produced in coda. This undoubtedly tied in with the fact that [Labial] was still generally weak in codas.

3. *Coda use*: As hoped, coda use increased because of the development of Labial-Coronal CVC structures and final affricates. The only missing codas were /l/ and /r/ (some of the time). Both singleton and cluster codas ([ts] for /ts/, /ks/) were produced, an unplanned bonus of targeting /s/.

Intervention Plan: Block 2

The second intervention plan addressed:

1. **NoSequence(Coronal. . .Labial)** (alternately, **NoSequence(Default. . .Nondefault))**
2. Onset clusters (tied to (1) above)
3. Nondefault features [+lateral] and [Dorsal]
4. Labial-Coronal sequences with labials other than stops and nasals in onset:
   (/f/, /v/, /w/)

The first two goals were combined:

NoSequence(Coronal. . .Labial) and **NotComplex(Onset)** (Clusters)

The more general **NoSequence(Default. . .Nondefault)** constraint was considered a particular problem for Harry. By addressing this constraint with labials, it was hoped that there would be generalization to non-nasal-nasal sequences. Specific contexts for addressing this constraint were CVCV words and CCV(C) words. Onset clusters were a goal for syllable structure, but they also provide (contiguous) consonant sequence contexts. In English, /sp/ and /sm/ are the only tautosyllabic Coronal-Labial sequences. It was felt that practice with those sequences might help facilitate production of other, noncontiguous, Coronal-Labial sequences. Homorganic clusters with coronals (/st/, /sn/) were included to help facilitate cluster production in general.

For the third goal (nondefault features), [+lateral] (/l/) was again targeted. The feature [Dorsal] (/k/) was introduced in codas (exploiting the rime cooccurrence constraint).

Because he was just learning to combine [Labial] and [+continuant], /f/, /v/, and /w/ were also targeted (#4 previously), in the Labial-Coronal sequence (to reinforce learning for that sequence).

Results of Block 2 Intervention (Approximately 6 weeks)

The most successful clusters were the Coronal-Labial sequences /sp/ and /sm/. Conversational production of /sn/ and /st/ was still inconsistent, in spite of the shared place of articulation. Further to the Coronal-Labial sequence issue, the first noncontiguous spontaneous Coronal-Labial sequence appeared (with an overgeneralized /l/):

zipper   /zɪ̵p /   [lʌpʊ]

Nasal harmony continued to persist, meaning that generalization of the Default. . .Nondefault sequence had not (yet) occurred.

Targeted nondefault features started to appear more frequently in conversation: [+lateral], and [+continuant] ([h], and [s] in clusters). [k] was produced in therapy contexts, primarily in coda.

Harry continued to have difficulty with sequences of complex labials (/f/, /v/, /w/) and coronals. In retrospect, it would probably have been wiser to target the complex labials in open syllables, where sequence constraints would not have been an issue. The feature cooccurrence constraints were probably sufficiently difficult for him without adding the sequence variable.

Follow-up

Harry continued with the same goals for subsequent therapy with further steady progress until he entered kindergarten,. In kindergarten he did not receive phonological intervention, although, after reassessment in first grade, phonological intervention was again initiated, primarily for /r/ (produced as [w]) and coronal fricatives. (There was variability in production of coronal fricatives: Either they matched the adult targets, or they were dentalized or lateralized.) Although there were no signs of labial or nasal harmony, occasional between-word harmony was noted for sibilants in connected speech.

CONCLUSION

It is encouraging when developments in linguistic theory can help motivate successful approaches to phonological intervention. Rule/process theories allow us to describe the phenomena we see occurring in children's speech in a general way that goes beyond the individual segments. Nonlinear phonological theory, with its focus on independent hierarchically organized levels, has been found facilitative for setting up phonological intervention programs. Constraint-based analyses such as OT represent another step on the way to explanation in phonological theory and they can also provide direction for intervention. In Harry's case, there were two major motivations for his pervasive harmony: sequence constraints, and (under)specification issues. Taking both into account in a systematic way and exploiting and considering other constraints of the system, helped provide a clear basis for an intervention plan. A process analysis would identify Velar Fronting, Stopping (or stridency deletion), Delateralization, Final Consonant Deletion, and Assimilation as processes to eliminate. However, the constraint-based analysis provided more detail about the Assimilation goal and how it related to the others. The constraint-based analysis provided useful strategies for intervention, in addition to goals. For clinical purposes, it was not necessary to construct elaborate constraint rankings with constraint tables, but it was useful to consider how several of the constraints interacted, and how they influenced each other.

In terms of Harry's progress over time, it was interesting that labial harmony became primarily leftwards rather than bidirectional, when he acquired more nondefault features. The high ranking of the **NoSequence(Default. . .Nondefault)** constraint in his system became apparent. Interaction of cooccurrence and sequence constraints was also revealing. Rime cooccurrence constraints facilitated development of certain nondefault segments in codas. On the other hand, feature cooccurrence constraints for [Labial] plus other features made Labial-Coronal sequences more difficult to pronounce.

OT is still in its formative stages, and we do not know in which directions it may be headed. The formalism and constraint names change frequently. For clinical purposes, however, constraint-based analyses can be used at least in a general way, as an effective addition to previous primarily descriptive approaches.

REFERENCES

Archangeli, D., & Pulleyblank, D. (1994). *Grounded phonology*. Cambridge, MA: MIT Press.

Bernhardt, B. (1992a). The application of nonlinear phonology theory to intervention with one phonologically disordered child. *Clinical Linguistics and Phonetics, 6*, 283–316.

Bernhardt, B. (1992b). Developmental implications of nonlinear phonological theory. *Clinical Linguistics and Phonetics, 6,* 259–281.

Bernhardt, B., Gilbert, J. H. V., & Ingram, D. (1996). (Eds.) *Proceedings of the UBC International Conference on Phonological Acquisition.* Somerville, MA: Cascadilla Press.

Bernhardt, B. H., & Stemberger, J. P. (in press). *Handbook of phonological development.* Unpublished manuscript, University of British Columbia and University of Minnesota.

Bernhardt, B., & Stoel-Gammon, C. (1994). Nonlinear phonology: Introduction and clinical application. *Journal of Speech and Hearing Research, 37,* 123–143.

Cole, J. S., & Kisseberth, C. W. (1994). An optimal domains theory of harmony. (*Cognitive Science Technical Report,* UIUC-BI-CS-94-02). Champaign-Urbana: The Beckman Institute: University of Illinois.

Edwards, M. L., & Bernhardt, B. (1973). Phonological analyses of the speech of four children with language disorders. Unpublished manuscript. The Scottish Rite Institute for Childhood Aphasia, Stanford University.

Grunwell, P. (1985). *Phonological assessment of child speech.* San Diego: College-Hill Press.

Hodson, B. (1986). *Assessment of phonological processes—Revised.* Danville, IL: Interstate Publishers and Printers.

Hooper, J. (1976). *Introduction to natural generative phonology.* New York: Academic Press.

Ingram, D. (1974). Fronting in child phonology. *Journal of Child Language, 1,* 49–64.

Ingram, D. (1976). *Phonological disabilities in children.* New York: Elsevier.

Ingram, D. (1981). *Procedures for the phonological analysis of children's language.* Baltimore: University Park Press.

Itô, J., Mester, A., & Padgett, J. (1995). Licensing and underspecification in optimality theory. *Linguistic Inquiry, 26,* 517–613.

Kent, R. (1982). Contextual facilitation of correct sound production. *Language, Speech and Hearing Services in Schools, 13,* 66–76.

McCarthy, J. J., & Prince, A. S. (1993). *Prosodic morphology I: Constraint interaction and satisfaction.* (Technical Report No. 3). Piscataway, NJ: Cognitive Sciences Department, Rutgers University.

McCarthy, J. J., & Prince, A. S. (1994). The emergence of the unmarked: Optimality in prosodic morphology. *Proceedings of the North East Linguistic Society, 24,* 333–379.

Menn, L. (1975). Counter example to "fronting" as a universal of child phonology. *Journal of Child Language, 2,* 293–296.

Moser, E. W., & Moser, M. B. (1965). Consonant vowel balance in Seri (Hokan) syllables. *Linguistics, 16,* 50–67.

Norman, D. A. (1981). Categorization of action slips. *Psychological Review, 88,* 1–15.

Prince, A. S., & Smolensky, P. (1993). *Optimality theory: Constraint interaction in generative grammar.* (Technical Report No. 2). Piscataway, NJ: Cognitive Sciences Center, Rutgers University.

Rumelhart, D. E., & McClelland, J. L. (1986). *Parallel distributed processing: explorations in the microstructure of cognition.* Cambridge, MA: MIT Press.

Smolensky, P. (1993, October). Harmony, markedness, and phonological activity. Paper presented at Rutgers Optimality Workshop. Rutgers University, Piscataway, NJ.

Stampe, D. L. (1973). *A dissertation on natural phonology.* Doctoral dissertation, University of Chicago. (Garland Press).

Stemberger, J. P. (1992) A connectionist view of child phonology: Phonological processing without phonological processes. In C. A. Ferguson, L. Menn, & C. Stoel-Gammon (Eds.), *Phonological development: Models, research, implications* (pp. 165–189). Timonium, MD: York Press.

Stemberger, J. P. (1993). Glottal transparency. *Phonology, 10,* 107–138.

Stemberger, J. P. (in press). Optimality theory and phonological development: Basic issues. *Korean Journal of Linguistics.*

Stoel-Gammon, C. (1983). Constraints on consonant-vowel sequences in early words. *Journal of Child Language, 10,* 455–457.

Gestural Phonology: Basic Concepts and Applications in Speech-Language Pathology

RAYMOND D. KENT

Gestural or articulatory phonology is distinguished from the other phonologies reviewed in this book by its assertion that phonological representation is in terms of articulatory organization as opposed to abstract features or other commonly assumed phonological units. Certainly, other phonological theories may refer occasionally to articulatory properties, but they do not place articulation at the base of the phonological system. What is unique about gestural phonology is that movements, or gestures, are at the core of phonological representation. Therefore, gestural phonology simultaneously addresses issues in phonology and issues in articulation. The intent of this chapter is to provide a brief overview of gestural phonology and to consider its implications for the understanding of selected speech disorders, especially neurogenic speech disorders and developmental phonological disorders.

GESTURES AND GESTURAL SCORES

The term **gesture** in gestural phonology is used to denote a class of articulatory movements rather than a single, invariant movement. That is, gestures are considered to be abstract and discrete specifications of spatiotemporal pattern. According to Browman and Goldstein (1992), gestures are "abstract characterizations of articulatory events, each with an intrinsic time or duration" (p. 155). This property alone makes gestural phonology rare, if not unique, among phonological theories. Generally, phonological theories possess only a notional time, leaving the calculation of physical time to phonetics or models of motor control.

The individual abstract representations of articulatory movements can be coordinated with the representations of other movements in an organization called a **gestural score** or **constellation**. The gestural score specifies the movements for an utterance. A phonological representation can be thought of as a score, or pattern, of composite movements, each having specified temporospatial properties. An important aspect of the gestural score is that the gestural units in a score may overlap in time. The possibility of overlap is an important property because it allows an interaction among gestures that accounts for a variety of phonological phenomena.

Gestural phonology erases the line that other phonological theories have tended to draw between phonology and phonetics or between phonology and articulatory representation. It also departs from typical assumptions about the linearity between linguistic units and speech production. This linear view undergirds what Browman and Goldstein (1986) call the "strict segmental hypothesis," which states that segments are defined by sequences of feature bundles. These bundles can be conceputalized as a matrix of features with nonoverlapping columns. Gestural phonology is not completely estranged from other theories, however, for it embraces certain principles of autosegmental theory. In particular, the gestural score can be related to an autosegmental representation. The gestural score that specifies the articulatory movements in an utterance can be redisplayed as tiers like those of autosegmental phonology. The chapter on autosegmental theory in this volume is recommended for readers who may not be acquainted with this phonological theory.

A primary assumption of gestural phonology is that phonological organization is rooted in part in the physical constraints of speech production and speech perception. Phonological structure is predicated on interactions among articulatory, acoustic, linguistic, psychological, and other organizations. This assumption means that phonological organization can be understood only through an appreciation of the systems from which it is derived and on which it is based. In most of the published papers on gestural phonology, articulatory organization has been discussed much more extensively than the other types of organization, and this review chapter will reflect this emphasis. However, the complete specification of the theory supposedly would draw on information from multiple domains. This potential for specification carries both advantages and disadvantages. Advantages accrue from the fact that the bases of the phonological system are ultimately explorable from empirical investigations and can, in fact, be implemented in a computational model. Disadvantages follow from the inadequacies of available information on the physical, physiological, and psychological processes of speech.

To base phonological representation on articulatory organization requires an adequate model of articulatory patterns in speech. To meet this requirement, gestural phonology has been developed in large part using a task dynamic model of speech production. (For a review of task dynamic models, see Fowler, Rubin, Remez, & Turvey, 1980; Saltzman, & Kelso, 1987). Because of the importance of this model to many of the papers on gestural phonology, the rudiments of task dynamics are reviewed here before considering gestural phonology per se. But it should be noted that a task dynamic model is not an absolute requirement for a gestural approach. For example, Kroger (1993) and Kroger, Shroder, and Opgen-Rhein (1995) developed a gestural production model in which the control parameters directly defined vocal tract constrictions.

TASK DYNAMIC MODEL
OF SPEECH PRODUCTION

General Aspects of Dynamics Systems Theory

Dynamic systems theory (also known as **task dynamics theory** or **action theory**) conceptualizes speech or any motor behavior in terms of the interactions between biomechanical systems and environmental variables. These interactions define a nonlinear dynamic model. The model is nonlinear in that it has several stable operational regions with relatively simple control features. One way of expressing the simplicity of control is to say that the system possesses relatively few degrees of freedom. The degrees of freedom problem is a major obstacle in accounting for the control of movement. Even relatively simple movements can present a formidable control challenge if all the actions in individual muscles and joints must be specified individually for every movement to be performed. But if several muscles or joints can be considered as a unit, then control of the unit is a simpler problem. That is, a system that appears highly complex when it is considered in terms of its individual components becomes a simpler system if the components are functionally linked in units.

The degrees of freedom problem, then, is solved by conceptualizing the system as being composed of functional groupings. This approach obviates the need to control each component of the system individually. Functional groupings have been called **linkages** (Boylls, 1975); **synergies** (Gurfinkel, Kots, Pal'tsev, & Fel'dman, 1971); **collectives** (Gel'fand, Gurfinkel, Tsetlin, & Shik, 1971), or **coordinative structures** (Easton, 1972). In dynamic systems theory, a major part of the control problem is solved once the appropriate coordinative structures are identified. These coordinate structures are task-specific, context-sensitive, and adaptive. They become a powerful and economical means of accomplishing motor control.

A further advantage of the coordinative structures is that they afford a convenient regulation of movement parameters related to changes in rate or total displacement. The means to this regulation depends on a distinction between the **essential parameters** and **nonessential parameters** of a movement. Essential parameters define the essence of a movement; that is, they refer to qualitative aspects of a movement's structure. The essential parameter for a bilabial stop is the accomplishment of lip closure. Nonessential parameters determine the quantitative aspects of a movement. These parameters are quantitative, scalar variations. Taking again the example of lip closure, nonessential parameters account for differing displacements of the lower lip in reaching bilabial closure because of changes in phonetic context, stress, or speaking rate. The interplay of essential and nonessential parameters in speech production affords strong advantages in movement regulation. The essential parameters can account for the phonetically distinctive aspects of movement, and the nonessential parameters can account for the effects of stress, rate, and other scalar variables that modify movements under the restriction of phonetic requirements.

The relationships among the components of a given coordinative structure and the motor consequence of the synergetic relationship are determined by **equations of constraint**. These equations specify how the members of the group can interact within the limits of a particular action and its environmental circumstances, that is, the task. The equations allow a principled variation in the actions of the components.

As already noted, a problem common to the understanding of many physical and biological systems is the degrees of freedom problem. The solution is to compress system complexity to a small number of degrees of freedom, sometimes called **order parameters**. These parameters are associated with equations of motion (dynamics) that are both low-dimensional and nonlinear. The solution to the degrees of freedom problem lies in examining the behavior of the system for **phase transitions**, that is, circumstances that introduce a qualitative change in the system's behavior. One well-studied example is locomotion of the horse. The horse's gait demonstrates phase transitions as it changes from trot to gallop. Phase transitions are examined to identify the order parameter that characterizes the pattern and the control parameters within which patterns occur. The equations of motion for a complex system can be used to identify **attractors**, or stable solutions in the dynamics of the nonlinear system.

Models of Gestural Patterning

One of the most recent directions in the modeling of speech production involves the specification of speech in terms of gestures, or bundles of gestures. The term gesture in these models refers to a family of functionally equivalent movement patterns that are actively regulated to achieve a goal relevant to speech. For example, taking the simple example of bilabial closure for [b] as a speech goal, the family of movement patterns could include various combinations of jaw, lower lip, and upper lip movements. A gesture includes many aspects of speech production that have been discussed under categories such as context sensitivity or motor equivalence. Concepts of gestural patterning have been proposed by Browman and Goldstein (1986), Lofqvist (1990), and Saltzman and Munhall (1989). These gestural solutions to speech production are highly compatible with the attempts to use gestures as primitive units in a phonological system.

Saltzman and Munhall (1989) assumed that the invariant units of speech are gestures that relate to context-independent sets of parameters in a dynamical system. The spatiotemporal patterns of speech are considered to be the product of a dynamical system that has two interacting levels: (a) an intergestural level defined by a set of activation coordinates, and (b) an interarticulator level defined by both model articulator and tract-variable coordinates. The activation coordinate associated with a particular gestural unit gauges the strength of that gesture in effecting the vocal tract movements at a particular instant. Gestures may compete in terms of their activation coordinates. Each gestural unit is associated with model articulator variables that specify articulatory movements and tract variables that specify vocal tract configurations. The tract variable coordinates pertain to **context-independent** gestural goals (e.g., bilabial closure). The model articulator coordinates pertain to **context-dependent** performances of a gesture. Therefore, a given vocal tract configuration can have various articulatory implementations, depending on the tract-articulator relationships that apply.

Activation of gestural units at the intergestural level accounts for patterns of relative timing and cohesion for a particular utterance. This level defines a currently active set of gestures, which in turn are related to events at the interarticulator level, at which the coordination among articulators is determined. Each gesture is related to a tract-variable dynamical system. In the computer implementation of the model, the dynamical systems are defined as tract-variable point attractors (or stable equilibrium points). The attractors are modeled as damped, second-order linear differential equations that permit the model to generate articulatory motions in an articulatory synthesizer. Early results are promising. The articulatory patterns are consistent with certain effects in natural speech, including articulatory compensation (motor equivalence) and coarticulation.

GENERAL PRINCIPLES OF GESTURAL PHONOLOGY

Articulatory Organization in Gestural Phonology

The basic elements of articulatory organization are the vocal tract variables, the gestures, and the gestural score. The last of these may be redisplayed in the form of tiers, as in autosegmental phonology. Vocal tract variables specify the articulators that accomplish speech production tasks. As such, the vocal tract variables may be considered as the task variables that are controlled in a task dynamic model. For example, labial closure, or lip aperture, is a task variable that involves movements of the maxillary lip, mandibular lip, and jaw. The bilabial closing gesture defines a specific goal for the tract variable of lip aperture. Hence, vocal tract variables are assembled into gestures that represent goals of speech production. A basic tenet of the task dynamics model is that a given goal may be accomplished by different combinations of movements of individual articulators. For instance, the gesture of bilabial closure may be accomplished by various combinations of lip and jaw movement. Gestural scores are the means by which gestures are organized to reflect the articulatory patterns of an individual utterance. Examples of schematized gestural scores are given in Figure 8–1 for the four utterances *add, had, bad,* and *pad.* Relevant gestures are shown for the velum (VEL), tongue body (TB), tongue tip (TT), upper and lower lips (LIPS), and glottis (GLO).

Tier Identification Scores can be redisplayed as tiers. Tiers are identified on the principle of relative independence of articulations. Articulations that are independent occupy separate tiers. Velic articulations are virtually independent of other articulations and therefore form a separate tier. However, because oral articulations of both the lip and tongue depend on mandibular articulation, labial and lingual articulations are represented on an oral tier. The oral tier has three subsystems: lips, tongue tip, and tongue body. Glottal function is relatively independent and has its own tier. One version of a tier organization is shown in Figure 8–2. The glottal, oral, and velic tiers are all related to a skeletal tier that defines the basic phonological pattern (e.g., syllable structure) for an utterance.

Articulatory tiers can be supplemented by other tiers to yield a more complete phonological representation. This issue is elaborated in the following section.

Other Tiers in Gestural Phonology

The articulatory tier, such as a lip tier, is only part of the phonological representation of an utterance. Additional tiers include: the rhythmic tier consisting of stress levels assigned to syllable-sized constellations of gestures; an oral projection tier that permits lip, tongue tip, and tongue body gestures to be projected on a single tier; and functional tiers consisting of vocalic and consonantal tiers (following CV phonology). The addition of these tiers offers several advantages only briefly noted here. The rhythmic tier is the means by which stress information is added to the phonological representation. Each stress node in the rhythmic tier determines the stiffness and constriction degree of the gestures associated with it. The oral projection tier is correlated with the sequencing of canonical units and with acoustically defined phonetic segments. The functional tiers accomplish articulatory overlap between vowels and consonants.

```
-------------------------------------------------      ----------------------------------------------------
VEL                                                    VEL


TB        [---------- wide pharyngeal----------]       TB       [---------- wide pharyngeal----------]
                                    close                                                 close
TT                                  [- alveolar -]     TT                                 [- alveolar -]


LIPS                                                   LIPS


GLO                                                    GLO        [--wide--]
-------------------------------------------------      ----------------------------------------------------
                                    add                                                   had
A                                                      B
-------------------------------------------------      ----------------------------------------------------
VEL                                                    VEL


TB        [---------- wide pharyngeal----------]       TB       [---------- wide pharyngeal----------]
                                    close                                                 close
TT                                  [- alveolar -]     TT                                 [- alveolar -]

                close                                                  close
LIPS            [- lips -]                             LIPS            [- lips -]


GLO                                                    GLO         [--wide--]
-------------------------------------------------      ----------------------------------------------------
                                    bad                                                   pad
C                                                      D
```

FIGURE 8-1. Schematized gestural scores for four words: (a) *add,* (b) *had,* (c) *bad,* and (d) *pad.* Gestures are shown in brackets for the velum (VEL), tongue body (TB), tongue tip (TT), lips (LIPS), and glottis (GLO).

Phase Relations

The vocalic and consonantal tiers are coordinated according to phase relations. Some examples of phase relations defined for a single syllable-sized constellation of gestures are:

1. A vocalic gesture is phased with the leftmost consonant gesture of an associated consonant sequence. The associated consonantal sequence consists of a sequence of gestures on the C tier that are associated with a given vocalic gesture and that are contiguous in the oral projection tier. This principle established the general phasing relation among vocalic and consonant gestures.

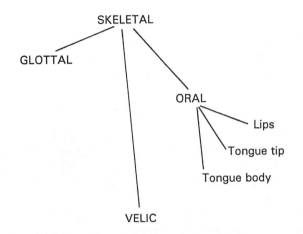

FIGURE 8-2. Simplified tier description. Gestures can be assigned to the appropriate articulatory tiers. Other tiers (not shown) govern factors such as rhythm, stress, and consonant-vowel coproduction.

2. The target of a leftmost consonantal gesture (the target being identified with 240° of a 360° cycle of movement) coincides with a point shortly following the target of a following associated vowel (the target being defined as about 330° of a full cycle of movement). In abbreviated form, the principle is

$$C(240) = V(330).$$

This principle specifies the phasing relationship between the leading consonant gesture in the C tier and a following vocalic gesture on the V tier.

3. The target of a leftmost consonantal gesture (as defined above) coincides with the onset of a following associated vocalic gesture. In abbreviated form, this principle is

$$C(240) = V(0).$$

This principle further fixes the temporo-spatial relation among associated gestures from the C and V tiers.

4. The constituent gestures in a consonant cluster are phased such that the onset of one (0°) coincides with the offset of its predecessor (about 290°). This principle can be abbreviated as

$$Cn(0) = cn\text{-}1\ (290).$$

With this principle, the constituent gestures of a phonologically admissible cluster are placed in a defined phase relation. (Kent & Moll, 1975, report timing data for the elements in a consonant cluster; their data show that closure for the first consonant in a consonant sequence is reliably achieved 10–20 msec before the release of the following consonant.)

Phasing of gestures can account for the control of movement patterns in phonetic sequences. Some examples were given by Kent (1986) for the phasing of velar and oral gestures associated with production of [k] followed by nasals or nonasals or the production of [m] followed by nasals or nonasals. The basic patterns of articulation are shown in Figure 8–3. The top part of Figure 8–3 shows the tongue raising gesture for [k] associated with two different gestures of velar elevation (a and b). The velar elevation labeled a precedes the tongue raising gesture, whereas the velar elevation labeled b is nearly simultaneous with the tongue raising gesture. The a phasing of velar elevation was observed for the [k] in *next*, whereas the b phasing was seen for the [k] in *camping* (for which the stop [k] is followed by nasal elements). Similarly, in the lower part of Figure 8–3, two patterns of velar lowering are shown in association with a bilabial closure for the nasal consonant [m]. The velar lowering labeled a results in velopharyngeal opening that basically precedes the bilabial closure (observed for the [m] in *camping*), whereas the velar lowering labeled b is essentially synchronous with the labial closing gesture (observed for the [m] in *Monday*). Note that the basic gesture of velar elevation or lowering is essentially invariant; it is the phasing of the velar gesture relative to the lingual gesture that varies with the phonetic requirements of the utterance.

Evidence of the gestural composition of an utterance can be seen in multi-articulator displays such as that of Figure 8–4, which shows movements of the tongue body, velum, and lips in a speaker's production of the sentence, "Next Monday morning bring three tents for the camping trip." The half-cycle sinusoids may be taken as idealized gestures from which the utterance is composed. Variable phasing relations can be observed for different phonetic elements. For example, in the three productions of [m], the first two have labial closure coincident with maximal velar lowering, but the third has labial closure that occurs with a pronounced raising movement of the velum.

Relevance to Problems in Phonetics and Phonology

A major attraction of gestural phonology is that it tries to account for a variety of surface phenomena with a relatively small number of under-

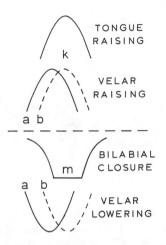

FIGURE 8-3. *Top:* tongue raising gesture for production of [k] associated with two different gestures of velar elevation. The velar elevation labeled *a* precedes the tongue raising gesture, whereas the velar elevation labeled *b* is nearly simultaneous with the tongue raising gesture. *Bottom:* bilabial closing gesture for [m] with two patterns of velar lowering. The velar lowering labeled *a* results in velopharyngeal opening that leads the bilabial closure, whereas the velar lowering labeled *b* is essentially synchronous with the labial closing gesture. See text for further description. (From "The Iceberg Hypothesis: The Temporal Assembly of Speech Movements" (p. 240) by R. D. Kent in J. S. Perkell & D. H. Klatt (Eds.), *Invariance and Variability in Speech Processes* (1986). Hillsdale, NJ: Lawrence Erlbaum Associates. Copyright 1986. Reprinted with permission from Lawrence Erlbaum Associates, Hillsdale, NJ.)

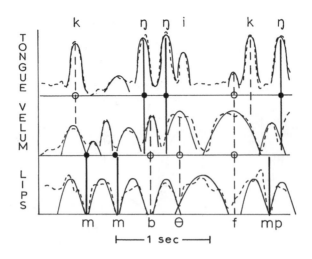

FIGURE 8-4. Movements derived from cinefluorography for the utterance, "Next Monday morning bring three tents for the camping trip." *Tongue:* vertical tongue body movement (upward movement indicates tongue elevation); *velum:* vertical velar movement (upward movement indicates elevation); *lips:* lip closing and opening (downward movement indicates bilabial closure). Actual data traces (slightly smoothed) are shown by broken lines. The sinusoidal half-cycles are approximations that highlight the abstract form of the underlying gestures. (From "The iceberg hypothesis: The temporal assembly of speech movements" (p. 239) in J. S. Perkell & D. H. Klatt Eds.), *Invariance and Variability in Speech Processes* (1986). Hillsdale, NJ: Lawrence Erlbaum Associates. Copyright ©1986. Reprinted with permission from Lawrence Erlbaum Associates, Hillsdale, NJ.)

lying properties. That is, phonological phenomena such as vowel reduction, place and voice assimilation, gemination and elimination of consonants, and elimination of aspiration all can be explained by assuming a representation in terms of gestural scores in which gestures may be variably scaled and phased with respect to one another. This is not to say that gestural phonology can account for all of the problems encountered in phonology. Its limitations have been discussed by several authors, but see especially Fujimura (1990), Kohler (1995), McMahon, Foulkes, and Tollfree (1994), and Tatham (1995).

Gestural phonology offers special advantages in accounting for articulatory variations in speech. For example, movement studies have demonstrated that coarticulatory patterns for velopharyngeal adustments and lip rounding can take the form of "one-stage" or "two-stage" movement onsets (Bladon & Al-Bamerni, 1982; Boyce, Krakow, Bell-Berti, & Gelfer, 1990). For example, opening of the velopharyngeal port in a sequence of one to three vowels followed by a nasal consonant may occur as a smooth movement that begins early in the vowel sequence and reaches its maximum during a nasal consonant (the "one-stage" pattern). Alternatively, the velopharyngeal opening may appear as an initial small aperture during the vowel sequence followed by an accelerated opening phase that just precedes the nasal consonant (the "two-stage" pattern). It has been suggested that these two movement patterns may be influenced by variations in the number of segments or by prosodic factors such as speaking rate or stress (Boyce et al., 1990). Similar variations in movement pattern have been reported for velopharyngeal movements by Kent, Carney, and Severeid (1974).

Another empirical observation that is more easily explained by gestural phonology than segmentally based phonologies is the occurrence of anomolous muscle activity recorded during tongue twisters (Mowrey & MacKay, 1990). The magnitude of activity frequently appeared to be graded for both inserted and original phonetic elements. The graded muscular activity could reflect scaling variations for gestures. The results described by Mowrey and MacKay present challenges to prevailing accounts of speech sequencing errors and to ideas about phonological–articulatory relations.

Similar behaviors may occur in speech disorders such as apraxia of speech, which typically is characterized by numerous errors judged perceptually as substitutions and distortions. Recent evidence indicates that speakers with this disorder may produce a highly complex pattern of dysregulation that is perhaps best understood in terms of phasing and scaling errors. This disorder and other communication disorders are considered in the following section.

APPLICATION TO SPEECH DISORDERS

Gestural phonology has not been extensively applied to clinical problems, probably because it is a relatively new theory and also because it is established on the dual foundations of a task dynamics model of speech production and some aspects of autosegmental phonology. Clinical implications of gestural theory in its broad form have been described by Weismer, Tjaden, and Kent (1995a, 1995b) for speech motor disorders. The following is a summary and elaboration of their discussion.

Speech Motor Disorders

Weismer et al. (1995a, 1995b) identified several features of speech motor disorders that should be taken into account in a clinically directed theory of phonology and speech production. It should be noted that motor disorders would fall outside the domain of most phonological theories because they exclude motor control issues. But gestural phonology, with its emphasis on articulatory organization and task dynamic modeling, has the potential to address these disorders. Because articulatory dynamics are foundational to gestural theory, disruptions of these dynamics should have implications for phonological representation. The common clinical features of speech motor disorders are: articulatory slowness, abnormal scaling of articulatory gestures, incorrect phasing of gestures, ineffective use of coordinate space, variability of speech production, segmentalization, and restricted adaptability to scaling variables. In addition, it is possible that certain disorders, such as apraxia of speech, could be explained in part by a deterioration of the gestural score. Each of these features is elaborated in the following.

Articulatory Slowness

Most speech motor disorders are characterized by slowness of articulatory movements. Although it is not entirely clear in a given speaker if the slowness is a direct consequence of neurologic impairment or compensation to that impairment (or both), it is relevant that many dysarthric speakers cannot easily increase their rates of movement, even under instructions to speak at a rapid rate (Kent et al., in press). The slowness therefore seems to be a basic dynamic insufficiency. If so, then the phonological representation is based on a dynamic system different from that of normal speakers. That is, the temporospatial specification of the gestures is inherently deviant. It is also possible that slowness may be one index of severity, especially in neurologic diseases such as amyotrophic lateral sclerosis (Lou Gehrig's disease or ALS) in which disease progression is accompanied by increased slowness of movement (Kent et al., 1989; Weismer & Martin, 1992).

Abnormal Scaling of Gestures

Scaling may be defined as the regulation of magnitudes of articulatory displacement as a function of time. In normal speech, gestures are scaled so as to reflect the coordinate space of vocal tract representation (Browman & Goldstein, 1988; Saltzman & Munhall, 1989). In addition, the scaling of gestures for a given motor score ultimately depends on the blending of individual gestures, each of which has its own scaling specification. Scaling often is abnormal in speech motor disorders, with both underscaling and overscaling occurring, depending on the type of neurologic disturbance. The disorders sometimes classified as hypokinetic (such as the dysarthria commonly associated with Parkinson's disease) are characterized by reduced magnitudes of movement. In contrast, some hyperkinetic disorders and cerebellar ataxia are often accompanied by excessive magnitudes of movement. In the task dynamic model used in gestural phonology, individual gestures are scaled in respect to the coordinate space that represents the vocal tract and the area functions for a given sound. Furthermore, the magnitudes of individual gestures are blended according to the gestural score. Errors of scaling are a means of explaining hypokinetic and hyperkinetic articulatory movements.

Incorrect Phasing of Gestures

Errors in phasing can produce a "sliding" of gestures that potentially alters the phonetic percept. Phasing errors may account for the frequent reports of coordination errors in disordered speech (Kent & Adams, 1989). As one gesture slides relative to the other gestures in a score, speech sound distortions or substitutions may be the consequence. In severe speech disorders, the phasing of gestures can differ markedly from that in normal speech. Kent and Adams (1989) give the example of movements of the velum, tongue, lip, and jaw in a child with cerebral palsy. This child produced abnormally synchronous articulatory movements (an "everything moves at once" pattern). Unlike normal control speakers, the child with cerebral palsy executed the velar closing gesture synchronously with movements of the oral articulators. Phasing difficulties also are implicated in apraxia of speech. Reports on this disorder point to dysregulation of the timing of various laryngeal and supralaryngeal events (Itoh et al., 1982; McNeil & Kent, 1990).

It appears that phasing errors may be variable in apraxia of speech, as discussed in the following section.

Variability of Speech Production

Many speech motor disorders are characterized by excessive variability of speech movements. Unreliable timing of movements has been suggested as occurring in several forms of dysarthria (Kent, Netsell, & Abbs, 1979; Hirose, 1986) and apraxia of speech (Kent & Rosenbek, 1983; Weismer, 1991). Faulty control of movement timing could be explained as deficiencies in the phasing of gestures in a task dynamic model of speech production. It has been noted that timing errors could contribute to errors that are clinically described as distortions and substitutions (Kent & Adams, 1989; McNeil & Kent, 1990; Ziegler & von Cramon, 1986a, 1986b).

Segmentalization

Segmentalization refers to a reduction of the typical coarticulation or coproduction observed in normal speech. The disordered speech patterns have the appearance of having been "pulled apart," or separated, from their normal overlapped pattern (Kent & Rosenbek, 1983). Liss and Weismer (1992) reported on qualitative characteristics in apraxic speech in which the variability in the onset of the major transition of the vocalic nucleus was interpreted according to a segmentalization hypothesis. In effect, the apraxic speaker has a highly variable latency in the onset of the vocalic gesture relative to the initial consonantal gesture of a syllable. The starting frequency of the F2 transition serves as an acoustic gauge of the degree of segmentalization.

Restricted Adaptability to Scaling Variables

Scaling variables include stress pattern, speaking rate, and similar modifications of the overall pattern of speech movements. These variables typically result in a scaling of the magnitudes of the component movements. For example, increased stress on a given syllable is expected to increase the magnitudes of articulatory movements within the syllable (De Jong, 1991; Kent & Netsell, 1972). Neurogenic speech disorders often are associated with a poor adaptability to prosodic variations. Stress contrasts may tend to be weakened, and, as noted earlier, adjustments in speaking rate are restricted.

Deterioration of the Gestural Score

The understanding of apraxia of speech has evolved to the point that motoric disturbances are now thought to be at least accompanying aspects of the disorder, if not central to it (McNeil & Kent, 1990). Apraxia of speech apparently involves a number of types of speech errors, some of which might be labeled as phonemic substitutions, omissions, or intrusions, but with others appearing to reflect essential weakness in timing or coordination. The severely apraxic speaker typically has a slow, halting, and groping style of speaking. The complexity of the symptoms may reflect a deterioration of the gestural score together with specific movement dysfunction. The hypothesized deterioration of the gestural score is consistent with the labored speaking pattern and with a variety of speech errors. It is also conceivable that an apraxic speaker cannot effectively scale movements relative to the coordinate space of speech production. This would result in a faulty preparation of the gestural score.

Developmental Phonological Disorders

The relevance of gestural phonology to disorders in phonological development should be prefaced by a few comments on what gestural phonology might have to offer in the understanding of typical (i.e., normal) phonological development. A useful starting point is Studdert-Kennedy and Goodell's (1992) paper, which argues for a gestural account of early speech in preference to a featural or segmental account. Of particular relevance to this chapter is the statement, "Finally, we must remark another process, difficult for a featural account, and important to our later discussion: the tendency for gestures to 'slide' along the time line . . . into misalignment with other gestures, often giving rise to apparent segments not present in the target word" (Studdert-Kennedy & Goodell, 1992, p. 9). The notion of sliding gestures may account for a good deal of the variability in early word productions. A child seems to produce a certain gesture as part of a motor sequence, but the sequence is variably timed from utterance to utterance. Depending on the timing (or phasing) relations, the sliding gesture may give rise to various phonetic effects. Because variability in the utterances of young children has been frequently observed, this property takes on special significance in accounting for speech development in children.

Gestural organization is especially well-suited to explain variability in utterance formation. Goodell and Studdert-Kennedy (1993) concluded from their data on gestural coordination that children make major advances toward the adult pattern at the age of about 3 years. Kent (1992) described other features of early motor control related to the emergence of phonetic classes and phonological patterns. These features were inferred from typical patterns of speech development and also from the patterns in phonologically disordered children. The motoric interpretations are compatible with gestural phonology and should be useful in formulating a developmental perspective on gestural phonology.

The prelinguistic emergence of discrete gestures in babbling may prefigure the gestures used in adult speech production. The babbling gestures may have a rather crude form that is refined during speech development (Browman & Goldstein, 1992). As such, gestures could account for some of the continuities observed between babbling and early speech (Kent & Miolo, 1995; Oller, Weiman, Doyle, & Ross, 1976;

Vihman, Ferguson, & Elbert, 1986). The evidence for developmental continuity is considerable, and it is therefore attractive to seek the roots of phonetic development in early babbling. Browman and Goldstein (1992) suggest that speech development in children also could involve the processes of differentiation and coordination of gestures. Presumably, the crude gestures used in babbling would give rise to a more elaborated set of gestures suitable for the phonetic requirements of the language. The appropriate coordination of these elaborated gestures would account for many aspects of phonological development. Hence, assuming that gestures initially appear during babbling, speech development could be based on the principles of refinement, differentiation, and coordination of gestures.

A major strength ascribed to gestural phonology in adult languages is the capacity of changes in gesture magnitude and intergestural phasing to describe a variety of phonetic alternations, including segment insertion, deletion, assimilation, and weakening. The same advantages may accrue to the description of phonological disorders. For example, some of the commonly described phonological processes may be interpreted to relate to changes in gesture magnitude or intergestural phasing as follows.

1. Final consonant devoicing is the result of an inappropriate phasing of the glottal gesture (specifically the devoicing component) with the oral projection tier. The glottal gesture reaches its target prematurely, thereby accomplishing a voiceless configuration before the oral gestures are complete. This phasing interpretation of a developmental phonological phenomenon carries the implication that a child's learning of proper phasing patterns will lead to the normalization of the voicing contrast for final-position consonants.

2. Epenthesis of a schwa in a consonant cluster occurs because of errors in intersyllabic phasing relation #3 (which, as noted earlier, describes the phasing between the vowel gesture and the leftmost consonant gesture) and intersyllabic phasing relation #4 (which specifies the phasing of constituent gestures in a consonant cluster). If the consonantal elements are not properly overlapped, the resulting motor pattern will be perceived to contain a brief vowel-like element, or schwa. The intrusive element will disappear as the child gains the necessary control over the intersyllabic phasing relations.

3. Stopping could arise as an error of scaling, that is, a child tends to produce an excessive degree of constriction.

4. Final consonant deletion could represent either an actual deletion of the phonological element or an insufficient production. The possibility of the latter was demonstrated by Weismer (1984) who showed that an ostensibly deleted consonant (that is, a consonant judged to be omitted by perceptual judgment) may be associated with acoustically discernable vowel-to-consonant formant transitions. The presence of this acoustic evidence indicates that the element is not completely deleted but rather is only fragmentally produced. This insufficient production can be explained by gestural phonology as a scaling error. It is not clear how other phonological systems would explain this phenomenon, except by attributing it to faulty phonetic implementation.

5. Gliding could be the result of a phasing error or a difficulty in achieving the temporospatial requirements for a stop articulation.

Although these examples emphasize articulatory or motoric events, it is conceivable that other phonological patterns are better explained in terms of perceptual operations or perhaps even operations that operate at cognitive levels. As noted earlier, the complete formulation of gestural phonology would include information on articulatory, acoustic, linguistic, psychological, and other levels of organization.

SUMMARY

This chapter has reviewed basic principles of gestural phonology and pointed to ways in which this theory may be helpful in understanding neurogenic speech disorders and developmental phonological disorders. The examples given only hint at the range of potential applications. The fundamental premise of gestural phonology is that a phonological system can be based directly on articulation rather than leaving the conversion of phonolgical output to articulation as a separate issue. This premise carries important implications for the study of speech and language disorders.

ACKNOWLEDGMENT

This work was supported in part by a research grant number 5 RO1 DC 00319-11 from the National Institute on Deafness and Other Communication Disorders, National Institutes of Health.

REFERENCES

Bladon, R. A. W., & Al-Bamerni, A. (1982). One-stage and two-stage temporal patterns of velar function. *Journal of the Acoustical Society of America, 72,* S104. (Abstract)

Boyce, S. E., Krakow, R. A., Bell-Berti, F., & Gelfer, C. E. (1990). Converging sources of evidence for dissecting articulatory movements into core gestures. *Journal of Phonetics, 18,* 173–188.

Boylls, C. C. (1975). *A theory of cerebellar function with applications to locomotion: II. The relation of anterior lobe climbing fiber function to locomotor behavior in the cat.* (COINS Technical Report 76–1). Amherst, MA: Department of Computer and Information Science, University of Massachusetts.

Browman, C. P., & Goldstein, L. M. (1986). Towards an articulatory phonology. *Phonology Yearbook, 3,* 219–252.

Browman, C. P., & Goldstein, L. (1988). Some notes on syllabic structure in articulatory phonology. *Phonetica, 45,* 140–155.

Browman, C. P., & Goldstein, L. (1990). Tiers in articulatory phonology, with some implications for casual speech. In J. Kingston & M. Beckman (Eds.), *Papers in laboratory phonology. I. Between the grammar and the physics of speech* (pp. 341–376). Cambridge, UK: Cambridge University Press.

Browman, C. P., & Goldstein, L. (1992). Articulatory phonology: An overview. *Phonetica, 49,* 155–180.

De Jong, K. J. (1991). *The oral articulation of English stress accent.* Unpublished doctoral dissertation, Ohio State University, Columbus.

Easton, T. (1972). On the normal use of reflexes. *American Scientist, 60,* 591–599.

Fowler, C., Rubin, P., Remez, R. E., & Turvey, M. T. (1980). Implications for speech production of a general theory of action. In B. Butterworth (Ed.), *Speech production* (Vol. 1, pp. 373–420). New York: Academic Press.

Fujimura, O. (1990). Towards a model of articulatory control: Comments on Browman and Goldstein's paper. In J. Kingston & M. Beckman (Eds.), *Papers in laboratory phonology. I. Between the grammar and the physics of speech* (pp. 377–381). Cambridge, UK: Cambridge University Press.

Gel'fand, I. M., Gurfinkel, V. S., Tsetlin, M. L., & Shik, M. L. (1971). Some problems in the analysis of movement. In I. M. Gel'fand, V. S. Gurfinkel, S. V. Fomin, & M. L. Tsetlin (Eds.), *Models of the structural-functional organization of certain biological systems* (pp. 329–345). Cambridge, MA: MIT Press.

Goodell, E. W., & Studdert-Kennedy, M. (1993). Acoustic evidence for the development of gestural coordination in the speech of 2-year-olds: A longitudinal study. *Journal of Speech and Hearing Research, 36,* 707–727.

Gurfinkel, V. S., Kots, Y. A., Pal'tsev, E. I., & Fel'dman, A. G. (1971). The compensation of respiratory disturbances of the erect posture of man as an example of the organization of interarticular interaction. In I. M. Gel'fand, V. S. Gurfinkel, S. V. Fomin, & M. L. Tsetlin (Eds.), *Models of the structural-functional organization of certain biological systems* (pp. 382–395). Cambridge, MA: MIT Press.

Hirose, H. (1986). Pathophysiology of motor speech disorders (dysarthria). *Folia Phoniatrica, 38,* 61-88.

Itoh, M., Sasanuma, S., Tatsumi, I. F., Murakami, S., Fukusako, Y., & Suzuki, T. (1982). Voice onset time characteristics in aprraxia of speech. *Brain and Language, 17,* 193–210.

Kent, R. D. (1986). The iceberg hypothesis: The temporal assembly of speech movements. In J. S. Perkell & D. H. Klatt (Eds.), *Invariance and variability in speech processes* (pp. 234–242). Hillsdale, NJ: Lawrence Erlbaum Associates.

Kent, R. D. (1992). The biology of phonological development. In C. A. Ferguson, L. Menn, & C. Stoel-Gammon (Eds.), *Phonological development: Models, research, implications* (pp. 65-90). Parkton, MD: York Press.

Kent, R. D. (1996). Developments in the theoretical understanding of speech and its disorders. In M. J. Ball & M. Duckworth (Eds.), *Advances in clinical phonetics* (pp. 1–26). Amsterdam: John Benjamins.

Kent, R., & Adams, S. (1989). The concept and measurement of coordination in speech disorders. In S. A. Wallace (Ed.), *Perspectives on the coordination of movement* (pp. 417–450). Amsterdam: North Holland.

Kent, R. D., Carney, P. J., & Severeid, L. (1974). Velar movement and timing: Evaluation of a model for binary control. *Journal of Speech and Hearing Research, 17*, 470–488.

Kent, R. D., Kent, J. F., Rosenbek, J. C., Vorperian, H. K., & Weismer, G. (in press): A speaking task analysis of the dysarthria in cerebellar disease. *Folia Phoniatrica et Logopaedica.*

Kent, R. D., & Miolo, G. (1995). Phonetic abilities in the first year of life. In P. Fletcher & B. MacWhinney (Eds.), *Handbook of child language* (pp. 303–334). London: Blackwell.

Kent, R. D., & Moll, K. L. (1975). Articulatory timing in selected consonant sequences. *Brain & Lanaguage, 2*, 304–323.

Kent, R. D., & Netsell, R. (1972). Effects of stress contrasts on certain articulatory parameters. *Phonetica, 24*, 23–44.

Kent, R. D., Netsell, R., & Abbs, J. (1979). Acoustic characteristics of dysarthria associated with cerebellar disease. *Journal of Speech and Hearing Research, 22*, 627–648.

Kent, R. D., & Rosenbek, J. C. (1983). Acoustic patterns of apraxia of speech. *Journal of Speech and Hearing Research, 26*, 231–249.

Kent, R. D., Weismer, G., Kent, J. F., Martin, R. E., Sufit, R. L., Rosenbek, J. C., & Brooks, B. R. (1989). Relationships between speech intelligibility and the slope of second-formant transitions in amyotrophic lateral sclerosis. *Clinical Linguistics and Phonetics, 3*, 347–358.

Kohler, K. J. (1995). Phonetics—A language science in its own right? In K. Elenius & P. Branderud (Eds.), *Proceedings of the XIIth International Congress of Phonetic Sciences* (Vol. 1, pp. 10–17). Stockholm: Royal Institute of Technology and Stockholm University.

Kroger, B. J. (1993). A gestural production model and its application to reduction in German. *Phonetica, 50*, 213–233.

Kroger, B. J., Shroder, G., & Opgen-Rhein, C. (1995). A gesture-based dynamic model describing articulatory movement data. *Journal of the Acoustical Society of America, 98*, 1878–1889.

Liss, J. M., & Weismer, G. (1992). Qualitative acoustic analysis in motor speech disorders. *Journal of the Acoustical Society of America, 92*, 2984–2987.

Lofqvist, A. (1990). Speech as audible gestures. In W. J. Hardcastle & A. Marchal (Eds.), *Speech production and speech modelling* (pp. 289–322). Dordrecht, Netherlands: Kluwer Academic Publishers.

McMahon, A., Foulkes, P., & Tollfree, L. (1994). Gestural representation and lexical phonology. *Phonology, 11,* 277–316.

McNeil, M. R., & Kent, R. D. (1990). Motoric characteristics of adult aphasic and apraxic speakers. In G. E. Hammond (Ed.), *Cerebral control of speech and limb movements* (pp. 349–386). Amsterdam: North-Holland.

Mowrey, R. A., & MacKay, I. R. A. (1990). Phonological primitives: Electomyographic speech error evidence. *Journal of the Acoustical Society of America, 88,* 1299–1312.

Oller, D. K., Weiman, L. A., Doyle, W. J., & Ross, C. (1976). Infant babbling and speech. *Journal of Child Language, 3,* 1–11.

Saltzman, E., & Kelso, J. A. S. (1987). Skilled actions: A task dynamic approach. *Psychological Review, 94,* 84-106.

Saltzman, E. L., & Munhall, K. G. (1989). A dynamical approach to gestural patterning in speech production. *Ecological Psychology, 1,* 333–382.

Studdert-Kennedy, M., & Goodell, E. W. (1992). *Gestures, features and segments in early child speech.* (Haskins Laboratories Status Report on Speech Research, SR111/112, pp. 1–14).

Tatham, M. A. A. (1995). The supervision of speech production. In C. Sorin, J. Mariani, H. Meloni, & J. Schoentgen (Eds.), *Levels in speech communication* (pp. 115–125). Amsterdam: Elsevier.

Vihman, M. M., Ferguson, C. E., & Elbert, M. (1986). Phonological development from babbling to speech: Common tendencies and individual differences. *Applied Psycholinguistics, 7,* 3–40.

Weismer, G. (1991). Assessment of articulatory timing. In J. Cooper (Ed.), *Assessment of speech and voice production: Research and clinical applications.* (NIDCD Monograph Volume 1, pp. 84–95). Bethesda, MD: National Institutes of Health.

Weismer, G. (1984). Acoustic analysis strategies for the refinement of phonological analysis. *ASHA Monographs, 22,* 30–52.

Weismer, G., & Martin, R. E. (1992). Acoustic and perceptual approaches to the study of intelligibility. In R. D. Kent (Ed.), *Intelligibility in speech disorders* (pp. 67–118). Amsterdam: John Benjamins.

Weismer, G., Tjaden, K., & Kent, R. D. (1995a). Can articulatory behavior in speech disorders be accounted for by theories of normal speech production? *Journal of Phonetics, 23,* 149–164.

Weismer, G., Tjaden, K., & Kent, R. D. (1995b). Speech production theory and articulatory behavior in motor speech disorders. In F. Bell-Berti & L. J. Raphael (Eds.), *Producing speech: Contemporary issues [for Katherine Safford Harris]* (pp. 35–50). New York: American Institute of Physics.

Ziegler, W., & von Cramon, D. (1986a). Disturbed coarticulation in apraxia of speech: Acoustic evidence. *Brain and Language, 29,* 34–47.

Ziegler, W., & von Cramon, D. (1986b). Timing deficits in apraxia of speech. *European Archives of Psychiatric and Neurological Science, 236,* 44–49.

Index